THE
CHEMISTRY
OF
HUMAN
BEHAVIOR

Herbert L. Meltzer

THE
CHEMISTRY
OF
HUMAN
BEHAVIOR

illustrations by
Francesca de Majo

Nelson-Hall/Chicago

Library of Congress Cataloging in Publication Data

Meltzer, Herbert L., 1921-
 The chemistry of human behavior.

 Bibliography: p.
 Includes index.
 1. Brain chemistry. 2. Human behavior. I. Title.
QP376.M525   612'.82   77-19195
ISBN 0-88229-177-7

Manufactured in the United States of America

10   9   8   7   6   5   4   3   2   1

CONTENTS

INTRODUCTION

If I were to formalize my long-term goals as a neurochemist, they would be to learn something of how the brain works, to describe what goes wrong chemically when it does not work well, and hopefully to specify the chemical intervention needed to make it work again.

In that sense this book might have been titled, "What We Think We Know About How the Brain Works." Its principal focus is on the brain as a functioning organ and on the incredible complexity of its chemical and morphological organization. But its particular focus is on the implications of such complexity for the capacity to obtain an information-processing system, packed within the space of just one skull, whose level of performance is well above that of any roomful of electronics we have yet been able to design. It is the tight packing that makes any animal brain a unique structure because of the clear implication that the significant structures within it are no larger than molecules.

To this end I have sought to describe in relatively simple statements what we know and believe about brain chemistry. I have omitted, for the most part, detailed discussion of how the knowledge was acquired, how strong or weak the evidence is, and who gets the credit for it all. This book, then, is clearly not for the specialist. Rather, it is intended as a progress report for the informed layman. Its goal is to inform where we think we are in the pursuit of detailed knowledge of brain chemistry, how this knowledge might relate to human behavior, and where further exploration is needed.

A large portion of what we know about the human brain is inferential since it is extrapolated from animal experimentation. It is the intent of this book to relate chemistry to human behavior; meeting that goal requires an understanding of neurochemical events that depend in large part upon knowledge gleaned from other species. Consequently, large portions of this book are devoted to chemical and behavioral observations of nonhuman subjects.

Since it is clearly not sufficient to write about what chemicals are present without defining their location, I have found it desirable to describe briefly the morphology and microscopic structure of the brain. In the same sense it has been necessary to couple descriptions of functional utilization of chemicals in the brain with a background statement of information theory.

More than in any other field of science, any book about the brain written at this time must raise more questions than it provides answers, for we are only now beginning to have the faintest idea of how the 10 trillion synapses and associated neuronal circuitry might be organized to provide those mixed qualities of intelligence and irrationality, hope and fear, and tenderness and anger that we recognize as human behavior.

PART ONE

Organization and Growth of the Brain

1

The Physical Structure of the Brain

AT INTERVALS RANGING from 45 to 90 minutes each of us, while asleep, enters a phase known as rapid eye movement (REM) sleep. The REM phase, which lasts several minutes, is recognizable by a reduction in muscle tone, a greater electrical activity in the electroencephalogram (EEG), and by the occurrence of dreams which appear to coincide in duration with the REM period. The pacemaker that apparently initiates these events is located deep within the brain. It is a small nucleus known as the locus caeruleus, and it is only one of many specialized regions that have been recognized as a result of careful anatomical study coupled with neurophysiological observation. The term "nucleus" as used here refers to a group of nerve cells, or more exactly, to a group of cell bodies of nerve cells. The term "nerve" refers to bundles of axons emanating from nerve cell bodies. A single axon is called a fiber. These distinctions will be specified in greater detail later in this chapter.

There are, in fact, two loci caerulei, located in each half of the brain. From outward appearances at least, most of the recog-

3

nizable anatomical features of the brain appear to be duplicated in the left and right hemispheres. Some neurological functions and some chemical entities are not replicated, at least not quantitatively; such differences will be referred to where appropriate in succeeding chapters. Bilateral symmetry is the most obvious of many features that are apparent upon even superficial examination of the brain.

A Rapid Overview

A systematic description of the major structural entities of the brain may be begun by starting at the location where the large fiber bundles of the spinal cord enter the skull. One notices a region, progressively thicker than the spinal cord, that is designated as the brainstem. A portion, a little more than an inch long, with a diameter of about 3/8 inch at the spinal cord end, widens to almost an inch at its rostral (forward) end. This portion, the medulla oblongata, is immediately followed by the pons, which is recognizable by the bulging mass of transverse fibers that constitutes its ventral (bottom) surface. The pons begins with a diameter of about 1-1/4 inch at its caudal (rear) continuation with the medulla and ends about an inch rostrally with a diameter of about 1-3/8 inch. The dorsal (top) portion of the pons, the tegmentum, contains a number of anatomically and functionally recognizable features, among which is the locus caeruleus.

A structure continuing about 3/4 inch rostrally to the pons is designated as the midbrain. A portion of the locus caeruleus extends into the midbrain. The cerebellum, a bilateral structure which is dorsal and lateral to the medulla and pons, is morphologically a much more complicated region. It consists of an anterior lobe having no recognizable bilateral symmetry, a middle lobe which is largely composed of the two cerebellar hemispheres, and a posterior lobe which has a median portion and two lateral portions.

The diencephalon (interbrain) is a bilateral structure each side of which is composed of a thalamus, hypothalamus, and associated structures. The basal ganglia of the endbrain are adjacent to the diencephalon. All of these structures are overshadowed in size by the cerebral hemispheres of the endbrain which envelop most of the interbrain and brainstem (see Figure 1-1).

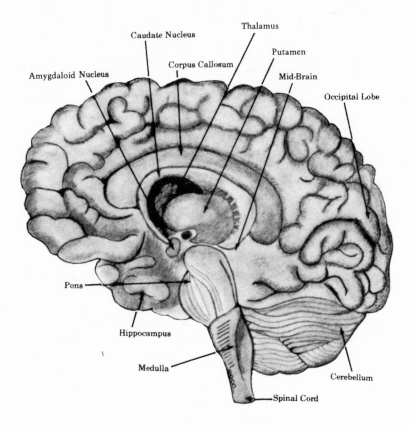

Amygdaloid Nucleus · Caudate Nucleus · Corpus Callosum · Thalamus · Putamen · Mid-Brain · Occipital Lobe · Pons · Hippocampus · Medulla · Spinal Cord · Cerebellum

Figure 1-1. Some principal structures of the brain. The view is of the right cerebral hemisphere from the medial aspect. Superimposed on this, in semischematic form, are structures of the left half of the brain, including cerebellum, brainstem, and some of the basal ganglia. The putamen and caudate are to be viewed as projecting from the plane of the paper closest to the viewer. They partially obscure the thalamus of the left hemisphere.

A More Detailed Examination

The surface of each cerebral hemisphere is folded inwards in many locations. Some of the folds appear to separate the surface of the hemisphere into larger regions designated as frontal, parietal, temporal, and occipital lobes.

A separation between folds is called a sulcus. A deep, extended sulcus is referred to as a fissure. A folded, convoluted region between sulci is called a gyrus. The frontal lobe, occupying about one-third of the hemisphere surface, is separated from the parietal lobe by the central sulcus and from the temporal lobe by the lateral fissure (see Figure 1-2). If the edges of the lateral fissure are retracted another region, the insula, appears below. A portion of the insula extends to the basal (underside) region of the hemisphere, where it meets the olfactory lobe.

Looking inward from the surface, each hemisphere contains a layer of gray matter, the cerebral cortex, which covers an inner fiber mass, the white matter. Within each of the two hemispheres there are fluid-filled cavities known as the lateral ventricles. These are two of the four ventricles within the brain, and the fluid within them, the cerebrospinal fluid, is continuous with the fluid in the central cavity of the spinal cord.

The roof of each lateral ventricle is formed in part by the corpus callosum, a massive fiber bundle most of which interconnects identical regions of the cortex of each cerebral hemisphere. Connections between differing cortical regions within each hemisphere are made by two kinds of association fibers. The first category—the intracortical fibers—connects cortical neurons within the boundaries of a gyrus, the boundry line being defined by a sulcus. The second category—the subcortical fibers—is further subcatagorized as either long or short. The short fibers dip briefly into the white matter to connect adjacent gyri. The long association fibers, located deeper in the white matter, connect different lobes.

An example of interconnections due to long association fibers is supplied by a fiber bundle known as the uncinate fasciculus, the basal portion of which makes a sharp loop around the lateral fissure (see Figure 1-3). The inferior (lower) frontal gyrus (a portion of the frontal lobe) is separated by branches of the lateral fissure into three portions. In the left hemisphere the two upper

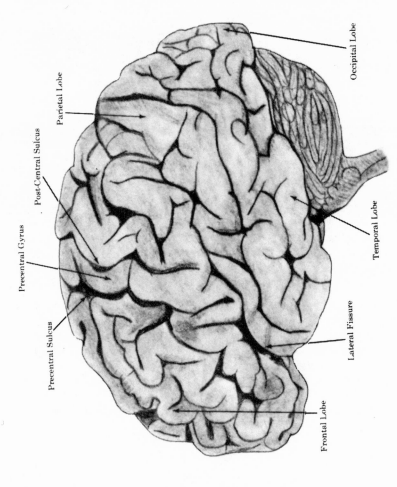

Figure 1-2. Regions of the left cerebral hemisphere, lateral surface.

Occipital Lobe

Parietal Lobe

Post-Central Sulcus

Precentral Gyrus

Precentral Sulcus

Temporal Lobe

Lateral Fissure

Frontal Lobe

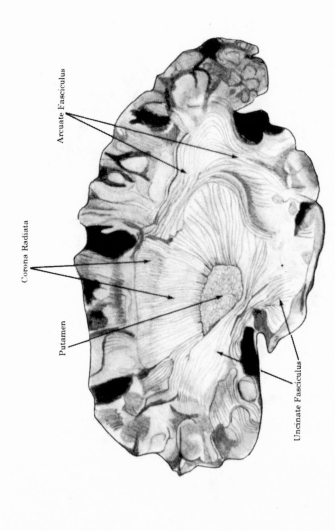

Arcuate Fasciculus

Corona Radiata

Putamen

Uncinate Fasciculus

Figure 1-3. Some association fibers. The lateral wall of the left hemisphere has been removed to show the under-lying fiber bundles. The corona radiata represents fibers arising from all regions of the hemisphere and converging toward the brainstem.

portions, known as Broca's area, are responsible for control of those muscles that give rise to speech. The posterior parts of the lower portion, the orbital gyri, are connected by the basal fibers of the uncinate fasciculus with the tip of the hippocampal gyrus, located in the medial (center and basal portion of the temporal lobe. The hippocampal gyrus and its inner extension, the hippocampus, together with the cingulate gyrus and other medial structures appear to form an inner ring in the medial region of the hemisphere, and they have been collectively designated as the limbic lobe. Together with some parts of the thalamus and hypothalamus, the designated structures are known as the limbic "system," which is under intensive study for its possible role in emotionality, aggressivity, and memory.

The basal ganglia are nuclei entirely enveloped by the cerebral hemispheres (Figure 1-1). Fiber bundles passing between the cortex and lower centers are intermixed with three of the basal ganglia, giving the group a striated external appearance. The term corpus striatum refers to this region which includes the caudate, globus pallidus, and putamen. The amygdaloid nucleus, a component of the limbic system, and the claustrum are the other two nuclei of the basal ganglia.

The thalamic region (the diencephalon), in close proximity to the caudate nucleus, is a complex of at least 25 nuclei which integrate and relay sensory information to the cortex, participate in limbic system emotional activity, integrate vision and hearing with somesthetic (body sense) input, modulate motor activity, influence EEG activity, and perhaps relate to the perception of consciousness and to the affective quality of sensory input. The hypothalamus is the major region for regulation of autonomic nervous system functions (thirst and hunger, sleep, regulation of body temperature, and others), as well as regulation of pituitary secretions.

The midbrain, just caudal to the thalamus, contains two important nuclei, the substantia nigra and the red nucleus. Both nuclei are important components of the extrapyramidal system (see below). Additionally, the red nucleus is a relay station in the interchange of information between the cerebral cortex and the cerebellar hemispheres. It is located in the tegmentum of the midbrain. The tegmentum is the upper part of the cerebral peduncle, a ventral stucture of the midbrain. The substantia nigra is located just below the red nucleus; both nuclei extend into the diencephalon.

The pons, caudal to the midbrain, is similarly divided into a dorsal portion, the tegmentum, and a ventral portion. The pontile nuclei are located in the ventral portion, as is a massive band of transverse fibers, the brachium pontis, which links the pons to the cerebellum.

The medulla, the most caudal element of the brainstem, contains on its ventral surface paired fiber bundles named pyramids from their cross-sectional appearance. Dorsal to the pyramids, near the junction with the pons, there is a nuclear mass termed the inferior olive. The nucleus cuneatus is located at the same level, just below the tegmentum of the medulla.

The fourth ventricle, at its caudal end continuous with the spinal cord, extends through the medulla and pons to the cerebral aquaduct of the midbrain. From there passage is continuous to the thin third ventricle of the diencephalon, which in turn communicates via narrow openings with the lateral ventricles of the cerebral hemispheres. Each ventricular roof contains a network of small blood vessels, the choroid plexus, that transfers water and certain solutes to the cerebrospinal fluid.

The tegmentum of the medulla, pons, and midbrain contains a number of nuclei at the midline, termed the raphe nuclei. These will be discussed in greater detail in a subsequent chapter, for they contain a large part of the brain's content of serotonin, a chemical transmitter (see Chapter 8).

Starting at the spinal cord and continuing through the ventrolateral region of the medulla, pons, and midbrain, there is an important network of nuclei and short fibers termed the reticular formation. Portions of this system extend into and through the basal diencephalon to the internal capsule, the thick band of fibers passing through the corpus striatum to the cerebral cortex.

The cerebellum receives information about position and movement of muscles (proprioceptive input), exteroceptive input (touch, pressure, skin pain, and temperature), and olfactory, auditory, and visual input, and interconnects with the cerebral cortex and all levels of the brainstem. It is thought to modify all neural activity, but it particularly affects motor coordination.

Nerve Pathways

Information flows via nerve fibers between various parts of the central nervous system, as well as between the brain and the peripheral organs and tissues it serves. The nerves are designated as afferent if information is carried to a designated area of the nervous system, and as efferent if the flow of information is from that area, either to another such location or to an end organ.

All information entering and leaving the brain does so by 1 or more of the 12 cranial nerves or by fiber tracts running to and from various locations in the spinal cord. It is well beyond the scope of this chapter to describe in detail the known paths, interactions, and probable functions of fiber tracts within the central nervous system. The following is intended only as an outline; the reader desiring a more complete account should consult a standard text in neuroanatomy.

Muscle movements, as for example the movements needed to turn this page, are controlled by two kinds of fiber tracts. The information needed to engage the page with the fingers is transmitted from the motor areas of the cerebral cortex, located in and near the precentral gyrus, to the required muscles via fibers of the pyramidal tract, so named because of the appearance of this fiber bundle in the ventral region of the medulla. There are over 1 million fibers in each of the two pyramidal tracts. Most of them run directly from the cortex to a particular location in the spinal column.

The larger arm movements needed to bring the hand to the page, continuing with the above example, are controlled by fibers of the extrapyramidal tracts. These tracts represent the output of the extrapyramidal motor system, originating from the basal ganglia. However, the overall activity of the system is dominated by the cerebral cortex.

The components of this system include the three basal ganglia of the corpus striatum, part of the subthalamus in the diencephalon, the substantia nigra and red nucleus of the midbrain, and portions of the reticular formation. Extrapyramidal fiber tracts originate directly from the reticular formation which in turn receives the output of other components of the system.

An incomplete and relatively uncomplicated representation

of the interconnections of some brain regions is shown schematically in Figure 1-4. All of the tracts shown are descending, carrying information from the brain. Ascending tracts, bearing information from the periphery, enter many of the regions shown and greatly complicate the interactions that may occur. A more extensive, though still incomplete, account of interconnections is presented in Table 1, for those nerves and tracts entering and leaving the medulla.

It will be appreciated that the specialized regions of the cerebral cortex, cerebellum, and brainstem can interact with each other in complex ways to modify incoming and outgoing information. Thus even at this level of gross morphology the structural diversity of the brain hints at the sophisticated functions of this organ. The study of the microscopic organizations of the brain provides a leap into structural arrays 10 orders of magnitude more complex.

Neurons and Glia

The neuron is the fundamental unit of brain function. Although there is no "typical" neuron certain structural similarities may be recognized among the various types. Each contains at least a perikaryon (cell body) and an axon. The perikaryon is not unlike other cell bodies in that it contains a nucleus surrounded by protoplasm which is in turn enveloped by a thin plasma membrane. One striking difference does exist, however: neurons, unlike most other cells, are incapable of replication.

The cytoplasm contains a number of fine structures, including mitochondria, microsomes, Nissl bodies, and neurofibrils. Mitochondria and microsomes, common to all cells, contain organized assemblies of enzymes, whereas Nissl bodies are dense regions of cytoplasm specialized for the synthesis of protein (see Chapter 2). Neurofibrils appear to be similar in structure to the neurotubules found in axons and, like Nissl bodies, are unique components of neurons.

The axon is a specialized protoplasmic extension of the perikaryon, arising from a region called the axon hillock. Its interior contains many closely packed neurotubules, parallel to its long axis, which are continuous with the neurofibrils of the cell

Cortex (1)

Caudate (2)

Putamen,
globus
pallidus (3)

Thalmus (4)

Sub-
thalmus (5)

Mid-brain
tegmentum (6)

Red nucleus (7)

Pons (8)

Cerebellum (9)

Substantia
nigra (10)

Medulla (11)

Inferior
olive (a)

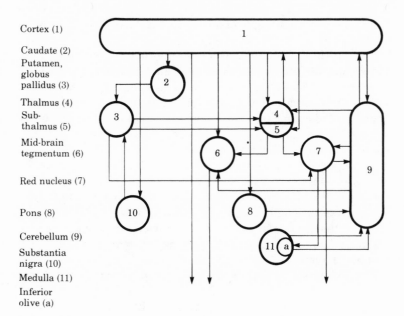

Figure 1-4. Efferent fiber tracts from the central nervous system and some regional interconnections.

Table 1

SOME FIBER TRACTS THROUGH THE MEDULA

Level	Origin	Destination
Nucleus cuneatus	Spinal ganglia	Thalamus
External cuneate nucleus	Spinal ganglia	Cerebellum
Nucleus of fifth nerve	Afferent trigeminal nerve	Thalamus
Reticular formation	Red nucleus, corpus striatum, midbrain tectum	Spinal cord and motor nuclei of cranial nerves
Lateral reticular nucleus	Dorsal gray column of spinal cord	Cerebellum
Inferior olive	Red nucleus, midbrain reticular formation	Cerebellum, spinal cord

body. The surrounding axoplasm is completely lacking in Nissl bodies, as is the axon hillock.

Axons in the central nervous system may be myelinated or unmyelinated. The myelin is a thick sheath, rich in lipid, which may envelop the plasma membrane of an axon for part or all of its length. At intervals of 1 millimeter or less there are pinched-off regions of the myelin, called nodes of Ranvier. The myelin is absent from the nodes. The diameters of axons may vary from 1 to 20 microns (millionths of a meter). Their lengths are quite variable, depending upon the cells from which they originate. In extreme cases an axon originating in the cerebral cortex may terminate in the lower part of the spine. Others may be only a few millimeters in length. Many axons have extensive branches. In general, the volume of cytoplasm contained within an axon may be much larger than that of the perikaryon, sometimes hundreds of times larger.

In addition to the axon the perikaryon may have other protoplasmic extensions, called dendrites. They generally contain Nissl bodies and their cytoplasm is not visibly different from that of the perikaryon. The dendritic apparatus of a single perikaryon may be very extensive, large branches leading to smaller branches to give a treelike appearance.

Most of the perikarya in the central nervous system possess dendrites and an axon and are termed multipolar; those without dendrites are either unipolar or bipolar. The bipolar neurons have axons arising at each end of the perikaryon. Unipolar neurons of the spinal ganglia have a single axon which divides a short distance from the cell body, sending one branch to a sense organ and the other to the brain or spinal cord.

Information flows between two neurons by way of a very specialized region known as a synapse. It is usually formed at the junction of the terminal end of an axonal branch with a portion of the dendrite or cell body of another neuron. The most common synaptic junctions are formed by side-to-side appositions of axons and dendrites (axodendritic synapses), axons and cell bodies (axosomatic), or axons and axons (axoaxonic).

Synaptic junctions have recently been the subject of intense morphological and chemical study. Figure 1-5 illustrates the major features of most synapses. The terminal region of an axonal

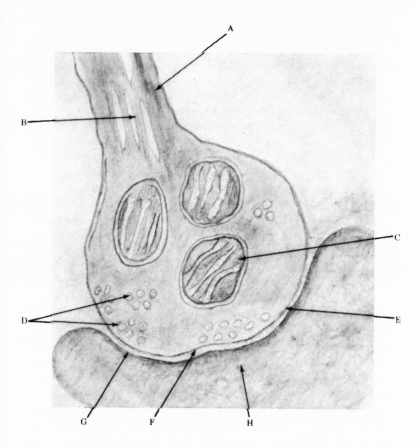

Figure 1-5. Diagram of an axodendritic synapse. A: terminal branch of axon; B: neurotubule; C: mitochondrion; D: synaptic vesicle; E: presynaptic membrane; F: synaptic cleft; G: postsynaptic membrane; H: soma of dendrite.

branch, called the presynaptic region, is characterized by the presence of clusters of discrete particles, known as vesicles, near the presynaptic membrane. Most vesicles are about 500 angstroms in diameter (an angstrom is 1/10,000 of a micron), although some may be as large as 1,000 angstroms. In addition to the vesicles the presynaptic region usually contains a few mitochondria and sometimes neurotubules as well.

There is a small gap, the synaptic cleft, about 200 angstroms wide, that separates the pre- and postsynaptic membranes. Electron micrographs of this region show a dense material to be present within the synaptic cleft. Dense material is also associated with the postsynaptic membrane.

The foregoing description of synaptic junctions applies to most of those found in the central nervous system, in cases where the nerve impulse is transmitted chemically across the gap (see Chapter 8). There are other junctions, however, where the transmission is more rapid. These electrotonic synapses have very thin gaps with a symmetrical structure on either side of the pre- and postsynaptic membranes. So far their occurrence in mammals appears to be limited to a few regions processing sensory information. The gap is about 20 angstroms wide and contains a network of channels between the adjacent cells as well as between the cells and surrounding fluid.

There are about 12 billion neurons in the central nervous system. The number of synaptic connections varies widely among different types of cells. A single axon may, by means of its many branches, carry information to many neurons. Similarly a single neuron may receive information from hundreds of different neurons. For example, the Purkinje cells of the cerebellar cortex have been estimated to have a synaptic surface area of over 200,000 square microns. In the cerebellar cortex of the rat there is one synaptic contact for every 3 square microns. If these two measurements are combined, it appears that there are at least 60,000 synaptic junctions for the average Purkinje cell. Pyramidal cells of the cerebral cortex, although occupying the same space as Purkinje cells, have many fewer dendritic branches.

With the more than 10 billion cortical neurons, and perhaps an average of 1,000 synaptic junctions on each cell, the 10 trillion interconnections make up a most formidable information system. Further complexity is added by the variation in size and extent of dendritic arborization of perikarya. Neuronal cell body diameters range from the 4 microns of the granule cells to the 100 microns of the giant pyramidal cells whose fibers form the pyramidal tracts leading from the motor cortex to spinal neurons.

The organization of neurons within the cerebral cortex provides still one more example of morphological complexity.

Three kinds of neurons are predominant. Pyramidal cells are shaped roughly like a triangle with the apex pointed toward the surface and the base parallel to the surface. A dendrite emerging from the apex, called the apical dendrite, extends toward the brain surface. Horizontally deployed dendrites (basal dendrites) branch extensively near the perikaryon. The axon originates from the base of the pyramidal cell and runs inward toward the center of the brain. Granule cells, which are much smaller than pyramidal cells, have dendrites emerging in all directions and axons that branch close to the cell body. Spindle cells are usually oriented vertically toward the surface. Dendrites emerging from the upper pole extend toward the brain surface; those arising from the lower pole branch nearby. An axon emerges from the center of the cell body and continues into the white matter as a projection or association fiber.

The arrangement of neurons in the cortex suggests definite layers. Closest to the surface, the molecular layer contains relatively few cells, most of which are either granule cells or cells with horizontal axons. Terminal branches of dendrites of pyramidal and spindle cells are located in this layer. The external granular layer (layer II) is a region of closely packed cells whose apical dendrites extend to the molecular layer and whose axons descend to the deep layers. Many of the axonal branches are unmyelinated. The pyramidal layer (III) is composed mainly of pyramidal cells whose apical dendrites extend to the molecular layer. The internal granular layer (IV) has many closely packed granule cells. There are many afferent myelinated fibers, some arising from the thalamus, in this layer. The internal pyramidal layer (V) contains larger pyramidal cells whose apical dendrites extend to the molecular layer and whose axons become projection fibers. Some of the fibers of the corpus callosum originate here. The deepest layer (VI) contains mainly spindle cells whose dendrites may extend to the molecular layer. Dendrites of the smaller spindle cells terminate in layer IV.

In addition to the neurons another kind of cell exists in great profusion in the brain. The neuroglia fill in spaces between neurons and are therefore termed interstitial cells. Astrocytes, one type of neuroglia, have protoplasmic or fibrous extensions that do not conduct nerve impulses. At least one process is attached to a blood vessel, while the remainder of the cell lies in close proximity to a neuron. Oligodendroglia are smaller cells which surround neurons or capillaries. The third type of neuroglia, the microglia, appears to be scavenger cells, whose size enlarges greatly in regions of tissue injury.

Earlier concepts of neuroglia as solely supportive elements are currently undergoing some revision. It is now postulated that they may have a more direct role in the processing of information, perhaps by regulating the electric field around neurons.

2

The Chemical Organization of the Brain

ONE WAY OF gaining insight into brain function is to attempt to find the location of the origin of a particular behavior. For many years the experimental approach to this problem coupled electrophysiological techniques with the ever-expanding knowledge of neuroanatomical details. Electrical stimulation of one area would be found to produce hind limb motion, of another, vocalization, and so forth. The result of electrical stimulation, however, is such that all synapses within the range of the electrical field are stimulated. Selective stimulation of particular synapses is not possible with this technique, but it is apparently achieved by application to a localized region of a very few specific chemical substances.

It is possible, in experimental animals, to surgically implant cannulae (small tubes) directly into specific regions of the brain. The animals recover from the operation and behave normally thereafter until the test substance is inserted into the cannula.

When acetylcholine (see below) was applied to a specific location in the lateral hypothalamus through such a cannula, a rat which had just satiated its normal thirst and hunger began to drink avidly. If norepinephrine (see below) was administered instead of acetylcholine through the same cannula, presumably to the same limited group of neurons, the rat chose to eat rather than to drink. At a nearby location, the anterior hypothalamus, application of a small amount of serotonin (see below) caused shivering and an increase in the body temperature of a cat. Norepinephrine at the same location caused a reduction in body temperature.

The effects produced are quite specific to a few locations. By exploring those regions of the brain from which responses were elicited, it was possible to trace neural circuits related to specific behavior. For example, 10 different sites in the limbic system were shown to be related to the thirst response.

Just as different substances applied to the same site produced different behavior, it has also been found that the same substance applied to different sites can produce strikingly different behavior. Acetylcholine, for example, produces circling movements upon application to one location in a cat brain, catatoniclike response at another, rage and purposeful attack at a third, and purring at a fourth location. The male sex hormone testosterone, when applied to the medial preoptic region of the hypothalamus, elicits maternal behavior (nest building and retrieval of infant rats) in both male and female rats. If applied to the lateral preoptic hypothalamus, it produces in both male and female rats a pattern of male sexual activity.

These examples point clearly to another aspect of brain structure—chemical organization. Neural circuits are activated by chemical transmitters (see Chapter 8), which allow the receptor neuron to "know" the source of the signal impinging upon it. Such discriminative capability is only possible if the structural and metabolic chemistry of the brain is highly organized. The chemical foundation upon which such selectivity rests will be the subject of the remainder of this chapter.

Structural Components

All organs and tissues, the brain included, are comprised of 75% to 80% water and an array of proteins, carbohydrates, nucleic acids, lipids, various metabolites, and inorganic substances. If one

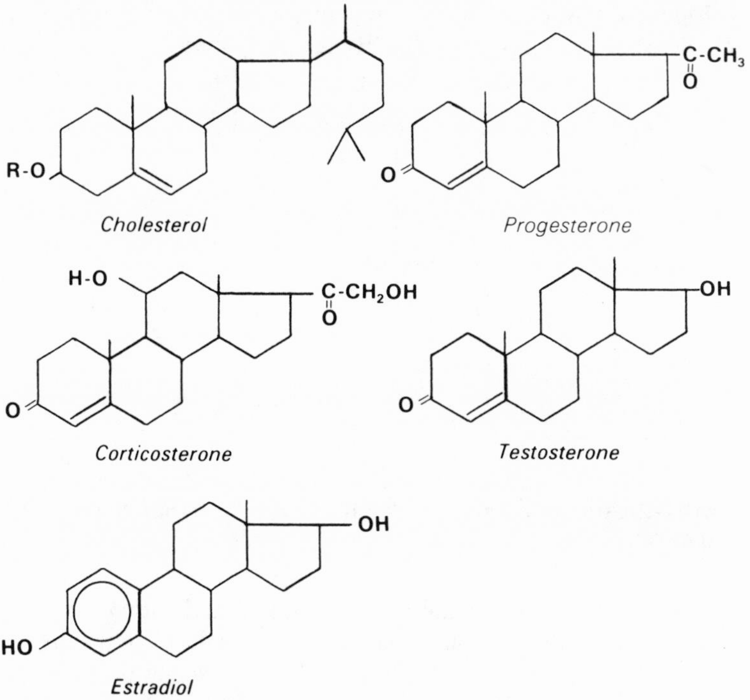

Figure 2-1. Some representative steroids. Note the presence of one benzene ring in the estradiol structure. Note that the "R" in the cholesterol structure may be either a hydrogen atom or a fatty acid moiety.

of these categories is to be chosen as characteristic of the brain, it is unequivocally the lipids, which make up over one-half of its dry weight. Cholesterol, phosphatides, cerebrosides, sulfatides, and gangliosides are classes of simple lipids, whereas lipoproteins and proteolipids are descriptive terms for two kinds of a complex association of lipids and proteins.

Cholesterol is one of many sterols in the body. Other substances based on the same steroid chemical structure are illustrated in Figure 2-1. Cholesterol is found largely in the white matter, as a major and characteristic component of myelinated fibers. Almost all of the brain cholesterol is unesterified (the "R" in Figure 2-1 is a hydrogen atom), in contrast to other tissues in which esters prodominate (the "R" is a fatty acid).

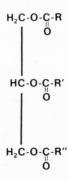

Figure 2-2. Structure of triglycerides. R, R', and R" may be different fatty acid moieties.

Brain fatty acids are almost always combined with other substances. The simplest of such combinations results from the union of 1 to 3 molecules of fatty acids with 1 molecule of glycerol (Figure 2-2). When, in place of one fatty acid in the triglyceride structure, phosphoric acid is introduced, the resulting molecule is a phosphatidic acid (Figure 2-3). Further substitutions on the phosphoric acid moiety lead to a range of phosphatides (Figure 2-3). One of these, phosphatidylethanolamine, is closely related to a plasmalogen (Figure 2-3), where the characteristic difference is the double bond between the first two carbon atoms of the fatty acid moiety. This seemingly trivial difference is of great significance to the brain's chemical structure, for plasmalogens, like cholesterol, are found preponderantly in myelin.

The third characteristic class of myelin lipids are the cerebrosides (Figure 2-4). They are composed of 1 molecule each of fatty acid, galactose (a sugar), and sphingosine. It will be noted that sphingosine can be regarded as a hybrid molecule. It contains the long array of hydrogen and carbon atoms (the hydrocarbon tail) characteristic of the fatty acids, but one hydrogen atom on each of its first three carbon atoms is replaced by hydroxyl (OH) or amino (NH_2) groups. (Compare with glycerol.) Hydro-

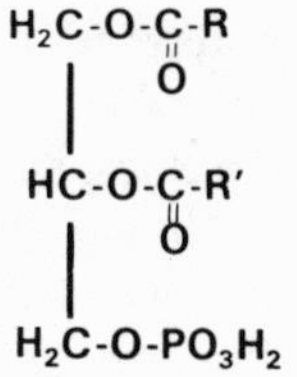

H₂C-O-C-R / O ... Phosphatidic acid structures

$$
\begin{array}{l}
\text{H}_2\text{C-O-C-R} \\
\quad\quad\ \| \\
\quad\quad\ \text{O} \\
\text{HC-O-C-R}' \\
\quad\quad\ \| \\
\quad\quad\ \text{O} \\
\text{H}_2\text{C-O-PO}_3\text{H}_2
\end{array}
$$

Phosphatidic acid

$$
\begin{array}{l}
\text{H}_2\text{C-O-C-CH}_2\text{-CH}_2\text{-R} \\
\quad\quad\ \| \\
\quad\quad\ \text{O} \\
\text{HC-O-C-CH}_2\text{-CH}_2\text{-R}' \\
\quad\quad\ \| \\
\quad\quad\ \text{O} \\
\text{H}_2\text{C-O-PO}_2\text{H-O-CH}_2\text{-CH}_2\text{-NH}_2
\end{array}
$$

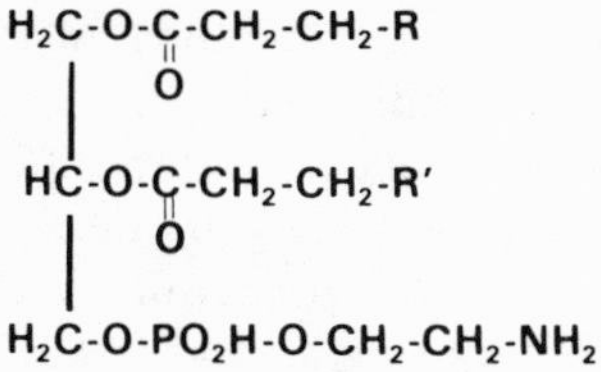

Phosphatidylethanolamine

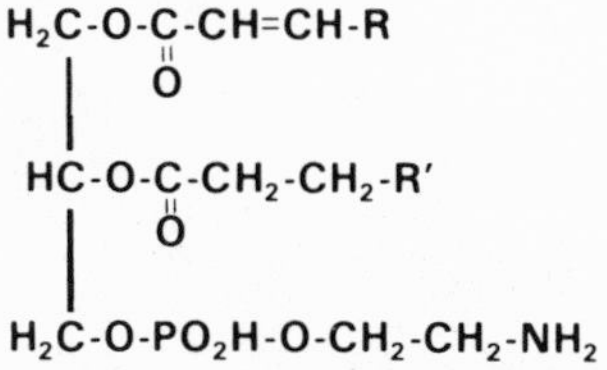

$$
\begin{array}{l}
\text{H}_2\text{C-O-C-CH=CH-R} \\
\quad\quad\ \| \\
\quad\quad\ \text{O} \\
\text{HC-O-C-CH}_2\text{-CH}_2\text{-R}' \\
\quad\quad\ \| \\
\quad\quad\ \text{O} \\
\text{H}_2\text{C-O-PO}_2\text{H-O-CH}_2\text{-CH}_2\text{-NH}_2
\end{array}
$$

Phosphatidalethanolamine

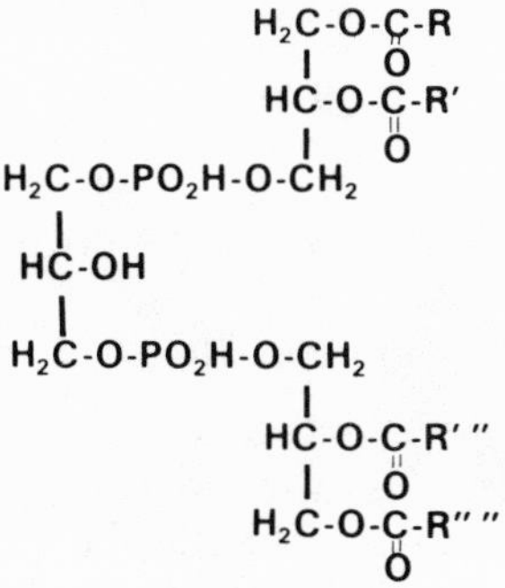

$$
\begin{array}{l}
\quad\quad\quad\quad \text{H}_2\text{C-O-C-R} \\
\quad\quad\quad\quad\quad\quad\ \| \text{O} \\
\quad\quad\quad\quad \text{HC-O-C-R}' \\
\quad\quad\quad\quad\quad\quad\ \| \text{O} \\
\text{H}_2\text{C-O-PO}_2\text{H-O-CH}_2 \\
\ | \\
\text{HC-OH} \\
\ | \\
\text{H}_2\text{C-O-PO}_2\text{H-O-CH}_2 \\
\quad\quad\quad\quad\quad\quad \text{HC-O-C-R}'\,'' \\
\quad\quad\quad\quad\quad\quad\quad\quad \| \text{O} \\
\quad\quad\quad\quad\quad\quad \text{H}_2\text{C-O-C-R}''\,'' \\
\quad\quad\quad\quad\quad\quad\quad\quad \| \\
\quad\quad\quad\quad\quad\quad\quad\quad \text{O}
\end{array}
$$

Cardiolipin

Figure 2-3. Some representative phospholipids.

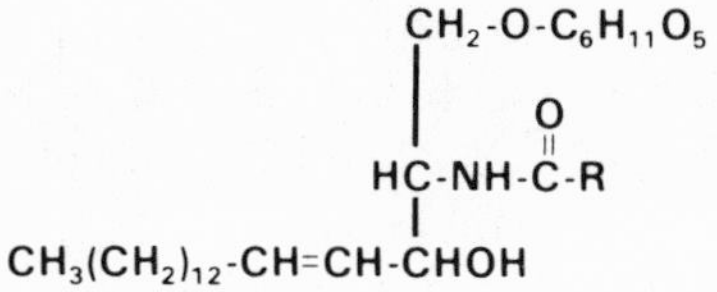

$$
\begin{array}{l}
\text{CH}_2\text{-O-C}_6\text{H}_{11}\text{O}_5 \\
\ | \\
\quad\quad \text{O} \\
\quad\quad \| \\
\text{HC-NH-C-R} \\
\ | \\
\text{CH}_3\text{(CH}_2)_{12}\text{-CH=CH-CHOH}
\end{array}
$$

A cerebroside

$$
\begin{array}{l}
\text{CH}_2\text{-O-C}_5\text{H}_9\text{O}_4\text{-CH}_2\text{-O-SO}_3\text{H} \\
\ | \\
\quad\quad \text{O} \\
\quad\quad \| \\
\text{HC-NH-C-R} \\
\ | \\
\text{CH}_3\text{(CH}_2)_{12}\text{-CH=CH-CHOH}
\end{array}
$$

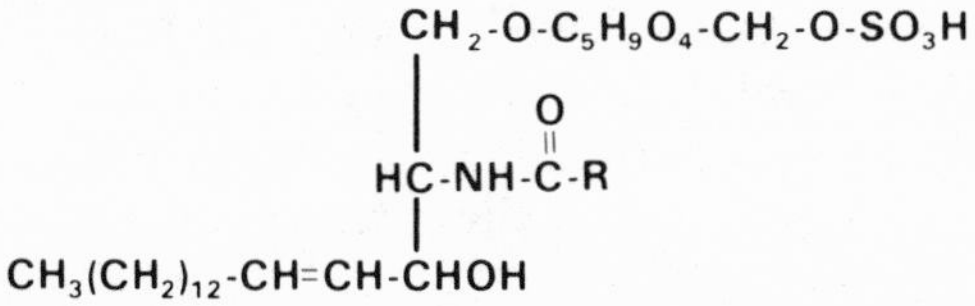

A sulfatide

Figure 2-4. Some glycolipids. The "R" is a fatty acid moiety. $C_6H_{11}O_5$ is a hexose moiety. In the structure of the sulfatide, the terminal carbon of the hexose is shown separately, with its linkage to the sulfate moiety.

carbons do not mix well with water and are termed hydro-
phobic. In addition they are good electrical insulators and do not
have a pronounced center of positive and negative charge in each
molecule; hence they are designated as nonpolar. Molecules with
many hydroxyl groups or amino groups, on the other hand, are
usually hydrophylic and polar.

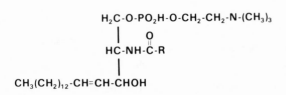

Figure 2-5. Sphingomyelin. The "R" is a fatty acid moiety.

Sulfatides, closely related to the cerebrosides, have a sul-
furic acid moiety attached to the galactose group (Figure 2-4).
They, too, are found more in myelin than in other brain structures, as are the sphingomyelins (Figure 2-5).

Gangliosides are polar, hydrophylic lipids considerably more
complex than those already discussed. The component moieties
include sphingosine, fatty acids, glucose, galactose, galactosa-
mine, and sialic acid (Figure 2-6). The number of sialic acid
moieties per ganglioside molecule forms one basis for their classification (Figure 2-7). They are found in particularly high concentration in most plasma membranes.

Common to all lipids is at least one fatty acid moiety. The
structure of fatty acids is based on the characteristic carboxyl
(-COOH) group found in all organic acids, to which is added a
string of carbon atoms, varying in length from 15-23 for the most
common fatty acids. These aliphatic chains may be completely
saturated (all bonds surrounding the carbon atoms are filled with
hydrogen atoms or occasionally hydroxyl groups) or unsaturated
to various degrees (Figure 2-8).

Arachidonic acid, one of the more unsaturated fatty acids, is
the metabolic precursor of another class of fatty acids, the prostaglandins (Figure 2-9). There are many different prostaglandins, existing in trace amounts throughout the body and having

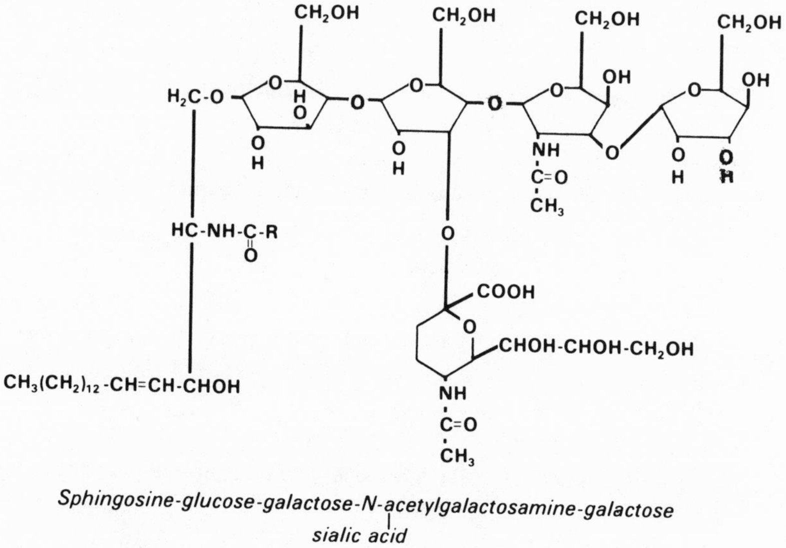

Sphingosine-glucose-galactose-N-acetylgalactosamine-galactose
|
sialic acid

Figure 2-6. A monosialoganglioside. The names of the moieties are diagrammed below the structural formula. The "R" on the sphingosine is a fatty acid. The combination of fatty acid with sphingosine is designated as a ceramide.

diverse hormonelike activities ranging from control of acid secretion by the stomach to promoting contraction of muscle tissue and participation in the processes occurring at synaptic junctions (see Chapter 8).

Proteins comprise about one-third of the weight of brain solids. They occur in high concentrations in the grey matter. Many proteins are structural in nature, occurring in plasma membranes as well as in the membrane boundaries of organelles such as neurotubules and mitochondria. Others are "soluble," occurring in finely dispersed form in the cytoplasm. Functional proteins include enzymes and perhaps those proteins that are implicated in memory storage (see Chapter 9).

There is a protein, apparently specific to neural tissue, that is presently designated as the S-100 protein because of its solubility characteristics. It is an acidic protein, a term used to designate

Ceramide-glucose-galactose-N-acetylgalactosamine-galactose
|
siälic acid

Ceramide-glucose-galactose-N-acetylgalactosamine-galactose
| |
siälic acid   siälic acid

Ceramide-glucose-galactose-N-acetylgalactosamine-galactose
|
siälic acid
|
siälic acid

Ceramide-glucose-galactose-N-acetylgalactosamine-galactose
| |
siälic acid   siälic acid
|
siälic acid

Ceramide-glucose-galactose-N-acetylgalactosamine-galactose
| |
siälic acid   siälic acid
| |
siälic acid   siälic acid

Figure 2-7. Outlines of ganglioside structures. Listed in order are a mono-, two di-, one tri-, and one tetrasialoganglioside.

proteins having an abundance of acidic amino acids (Figure 2-10). Basic proteins (those having an abundance of diamino acids) are also found in the brain.

Protein synthesis in the brain, no less than in other tissues, is directed by ribonucleic acids (RNA), which in turn are synthe-

$CH_3(CH_2)_{16}COOH$

Stearic acid

$CH_3(CH_2)_{22}COOH$

Lignoceric acid

$CH_3(CH_2)_4\text{-}CH=CH\text{-}CH_2\text{-}CH=CH\text{-}CH_2\text{-}CH=CH\text{-}CH_2\text{-}CH=CH\text{-}(CH_2)_3\text{-}COOH$

Arachidonic acid

Figure 2-8. Some fatty acid structures.

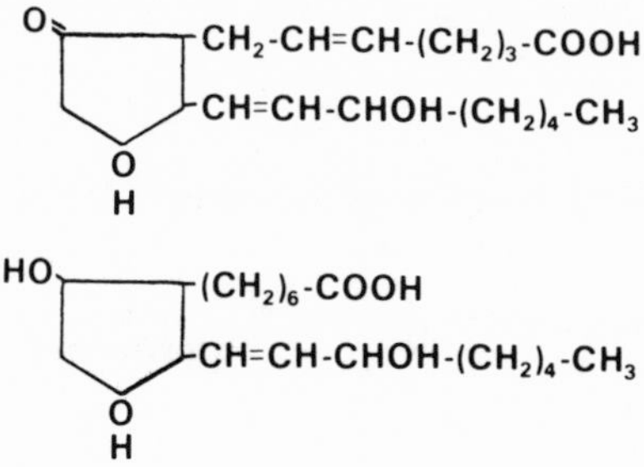

Figure 2-9. Some prostaglandins. Above, prostaglandin E_2 and, below, prostaglandin F_1-alpha.

sized according to master templates genetically transmitted by desoxyribonucleic acids (DNA). These substances are aggregates of nucleotides (Figure 2-11). One of these, adenosinetriphosphate (ATP) is a major source of chemical energy for a large variety of biochemical reactions. Its cyclized derivative, cyclic 3′, 5′-adenosine monophosphate, exists in the brain at about 1/1,000 the concentration of ATP, but it is strongly implicated as a mediator of hormonal actions in brain and many tissues (see Figure 2-12).

Carbohydrates in the brain include the glucose and galactose moieties of lipids, ribose of RNA and desoxyribose of

HOOC-CH$_2$-CH$_2$-CH-COOH
                     NH$_2$
Glutamic acid

HOOC-CH$_2$-CH-COOH
                  NH$_2$
Aspartic acid

HOOC-CH$_2$-CH-COOH
                  NH
                  C=O
                  CH$_3$

N-acetyl aspartic acid

Figure 2-10. Some acidic amino acids found in the brain.

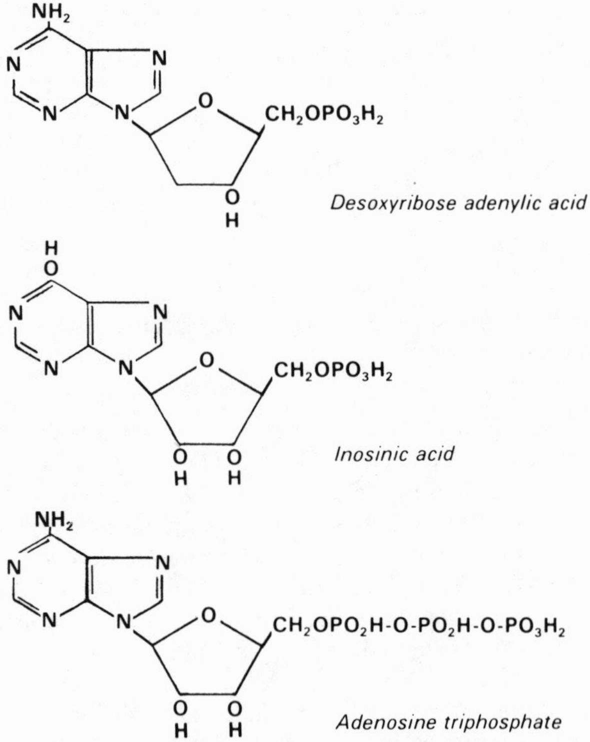

Desoxyribose adenylic acid

Inosinic acid

Adenosine triphosphate

Figure 2-11. Some nucleotides. The fused rings are derivatives of purine.

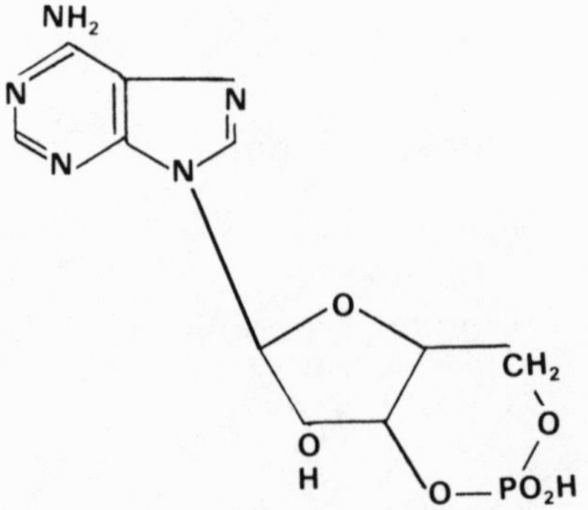

Figure 2-12. Cyclic AMP.

DNA, amino sugars of gangliosides, the phosphorylated sugars that occur during metabolic transformations, and a small amount of glycogen. The glycogen is a reserve energy pool, although most of the energy requirements of the brain are dependent upon transfer of glucose from the circulating blood.

Energy Flow Through the Brain

Although the weight of the brain is less than 2% of that of the remainder of the body, it requires 10% to 20% of the total energy intake in order to be able to function at all. The flow of energy to all organs and tissues of the body begins with ingestion of foods and inhalation of oxygen. The end result, catabolic conversion to carbon dioxide, water, urea, and small amounts of other substances, can be compared quantitatively with the oxygen intake.

The measurement known as respiratory quotient (carbon dioxide produced divided by oxygen consumed) can be carried out easily in experimental subjects. The respiratory quotient (R.Q.) arising from catabolism of a particular food is readily predicted from its chemical composition. Thus an R.Q. of 1.0 is obtained from carbohydrates and about 0.7 from simple fats. For many years it has been known that the average R.Q. of the brain is close to 1.0; hence it was concluded that a carbohydrate, specifically glucose, was its principal energy source. It is now known that the direct, instantaneous energy needs of the brain can be supplied by lipids, although ultimately the energy as well as the carbon atoms of glucose are required to restore the lipid content.

Before any substance can enter the brain it must pass what has come to be known as the blood-brain barriers. These are systems of selective permeability or selective transport thought to be associated with the astroglia. The selectivity of the barrier may be illustrated with glutamic acid, which does not pass the barrier, and glutamine, which does (Figure 2-13).

Glucose readily enters the brain if present in sufficient concentration in the bloodstream. As is true of other tissues, enzymes present in the brain convert glucose by a ten-step process known as glycolysis into pyruvic acid. At this stage two pathways are open. One effected by the enzyme lactic dehydrogenase (LDH) converts pyruvic acid to lactic acid. The second pathway of pyruvic acid metabolism leads to acetyl coenzyme A, which in

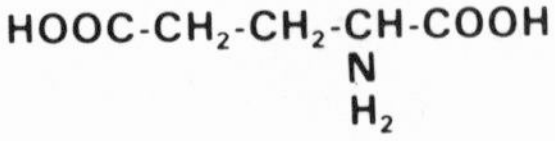

$$HOOC\text{-}CH_2\text{-}CH_2\text{-}CH\text{-}COOH$$
$$\underset{H_2}{N}$$

Glutamic acid

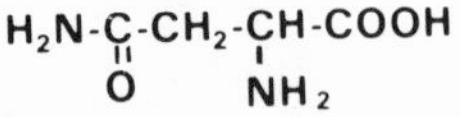

$$H_2N\text{-}\underset{O}{C}\text{-}CH_2\text{-}\underset{NH_2}{CH}\text{-}COOH$$

Glutamine

Figure 2-13. Substances impermeable and permeable to the blood-brain barrier.

turn can participate in two other sequences. One of these, the synthetic pathway, utilizes the acetyl group for the resynthesis of lipids and other substances. The second, oxidative phosphorylation through the tricarboxylic acid cycle route, utilizes inorganic phosphate and results in the formation of carbon dioxide and the energy-rich compound, ATP. A balance in the divergent pathways of synthesis and oxidative phosphorylation is in part under the indirect control of ATP. A deficiency of this substance is coupled with an increase in its associated nucleotide, ADP, which stimulates an essential enzyme of the cycle. Thus the oxidative phosphorylation pathway is regulated directly by ADP. The sum of both pathways depends upon a group of enzymes known as kinases, which add phosphate moieties to glucose and other intermediates. The three kinases are inhibited by excess ATP; the excess is recognized in situ by means of the local magnesium concentration. ATP, combined with magnesium, is not inhibitory. When there is more ATP than magnesium present the free ATP inhibits the kinases. Regulation of the activity of a metabolic pathway by means of interaction of the end products with an essential enzyme in the series is known as feedback inhibition; it is a common biological mechanism for maintaining the quantities of critical substances within narrow limits. The feedback controls outlined above are only a few of many that operate to regulate the metabolic utilization of glucose. The overall pathways of glucose metabolism are outlined in Figure 2-14.

Glutamic acid, an amino acid which is synthesized in the brain indirectly from glucose and directly from alpha ketoglutaric acid, reaches concentrations about 100 times higher than that

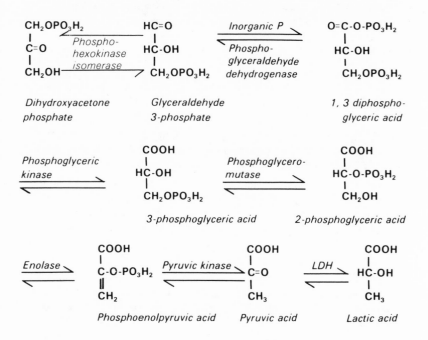

Figure 2.14. Some steps in glycolysis.

of most other amino acids in the brain. It is converted by an enzyme called glutamic decarboxylase to gamma aminobutyric acid (GABA). A transaminase removes ammonia from GABA and the product, succinic semialdehyde, is oxidized by a dehydrogenase and further converted to succinyl coenzyme A. This reaction sequence from alpha ketoglutaric acid to succinyl coenzyme A is known as the GABA shunt (Figure 2-15). All of these substances can supply substantial energy when further metabolized. In addition GABA is belived to be an inhibitory neurotransmitter (Chapter 8).

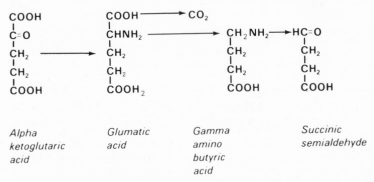

Alpha ketoglutaric acid   *Glumatic acid*   *Gamma amino butyric acid*   *Succinic semialdehyde*

Figure 2-15. The GABA shunt.

In addition to glutamic acid and its derivatives, N-acetyl aspartic acid also exists in the brain in a much higher concentration than in any other part of the body. All other amino acids are present in much lower concentration and are presumed to be incorporated into proteins upon demand. Control of protein synthesis starts with the DNA-directed formation of messenger RNA, which is then transported from the cell nucleus to ribosomes. The structures identified by histologists as Nissl bodies (Chapter 1) are apparently ribosomes, which can be obtained experimentally by removing the membranes from microsomes. Another species of RNA, transfer RNA, combined with amino acids, reacts at specific locations in the ribosome to progressively construct a particular protein molecule.

Many neuronal proteins are formed in this manner in the perikaryon. Some are required at locations in the axon a considerable distance from the site of synthesis. They are transported along the axon by a process known as axoplasmic flow, in which a continuous movement of cytoplasm takes place from the perikaryon toward the axon terminals. The rates of movement of specific substances have been found to vary from as little as 1/32 inch per day to more than 1 foot per day. Most of the "soluble" proteins are transported at the slow rate; some amino acids, phospholipids, and catecholamines (Chapter 8) are transported at the fast rate.

Thus the flow of energy through the brain starts with the selective entrance of glucose and other substances through the blood-brain barrier and continues with the generation of ATP and the synthesis of proteins and other substances in the perikaryon, followed by transport down the axon toward its terminals at varying rates. The fast rate requires the expenditure of energy, adding still another dimension to the possible variations in the chemical structure of the brain.

Intracellular Localizations

The nucleus is the site of most of the neuronal DNA and of histones (basic proteins) as well. Control of the expression of the genetic information of DNA is thought to depend upon interaction with histones. Synthesis of RNA in the nucleus depends upon the nuclear enzyme, RNA polymerase. An enzyme coupling two mononucleotides to form dinucleotides is also present. In addition to the histones, acidic proteins also occur in the nucleus.

The usual laboratory procedures for studying portions of the neuron result in partially purified fractions, obtained from a great many neurons. The following account of substances thought to be associated with specific neuronal regions may need revision as newer techniques lead to better purifications.

Microsomes are abundant in the cytoplasm surrounding the nucleus. They are composed of an inner ribosomal region, which contains RNA and enzymes of protein synthesis, and a boundary membrane. The more than 16 different proteins in the membrane comprise about half of its solid weight; in addition there is a relatively high concentration of gangliosides (about 15 times the average brain concentration), cholesterol, and phospholipids. The fatty acid composition of microsomal membranes differs from that of other membrane structures, in that more than 80% is accounted for by palmitic and oleic acids. Microsomal membranes contain a number of enzymes, among which ATP-ase and cholinesterase predominate. There are also enzymes of the electron transport system which are not found in significant amounts in other membranes such as the outer membrane of the perikaryon.

Throughout the cytoplasm there are a large number of rodlike structures called mitochondria. In a rat brain the average perikaryon contains about 1,300 mitochondria. A few are found in the axon and one or two are present in each of the many terminal branches of axons. They are the principal sites of oxidative phosphorylation; additionally, they may synthesize some structural proteins. Mitochondrial membranes contain about 20 proteins, the quantitative pattern of which is different from that obtained from nerve terminal membranes. Their lipid composition is strikingly different from that of other intracellular organelles, in that they are almost devoid of cerebrosides and gangliosides. Of the phospholipids, which predominate, 40% are lecithins, 20% phosphatidylethanolamine, 10% phosphatidalethanolamine, and 10% cardiolipin. The membrane proteins comprise 40% of the solids; many are associated with lipids as lipoproteins.

Many of the mitochondrial proteins are enzymes required for oxidative phosphorylation. More than half of the neuronal hexokinase is located in the mitochondria. Two enzymes, succinic dehydrogenase (SDH) and monoamine oxidase (MAO), are almost entirely present in mitochondria. MAO, an enzyme which removes the amine moiety from the transmitter amines (Chapter 8), is present in five different states of molecular conformation, all of which are associated with phospholipids. The enzymic activity appears to be increased by progesterone, which is also found in mitochondria.

Cobalamine (Vitamin B_{12}) is a coenzyme for several important reactions, including the conversion of methylmalonic acid to succinic acid. Methylmalonic acid is formed during the catabolism of the amino acid valine and from the biotin-dependent enzymatic combination of carbon dioxide with propionic acid. The amino acids isoleucine, methionine, and threonine, fatty acids with an odd number of carbon atoms, and the side chain of cholesterol are the principal sources of propionic acid. Succinic acid, once formed, is further metabolized through the tricarboxylic acid cycle (see Figure 2-16). Half of the neuronal B_{12} is

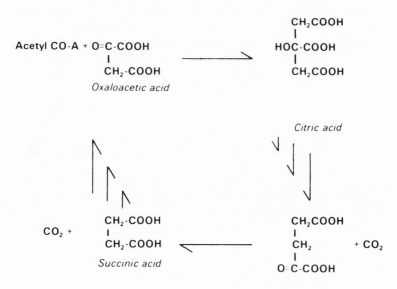

Figure 2-16. Some steps in the tricarboxylic acid cycle.

located in mitochondria. Lack of B_{12} in pernicious anemia is sometimes associated with psychosis and reduced EEG activity. Since B_{12} therapy can restore EEG function before it increases red blood cell function there is good reason to believe that adequate B_{12} is important for normal brain function.

Axons are distinguished chemically from dendrites and perikarya by a lack of ribosomes, by the globular proteins of the neurotubules which bind colchicine, and, when myelinated, by the characteristic chemical composition of myelin. The lipid composition of myelin has already been discussed. Of the protein contained in myelin, 60% occurs as proteolipid protein. This class of proteins is distinguished from other proteins by a low content of basic and acidic amino acids. Lipids and proteins in myelin appear to be arranged in concentric layers, with an inner protein layer followed by two lipid layers and an outer protein layer. When the myelin sheath is thick the pattern may be repeated several times.

The synaptic region that terminates an axonal branch has a distinctive chemical composition based on its function as a reservoir for transmitters. In the laboratory process of isolating it from other regions the nerve ending is pinched off to form an artificial particle called a synaptosome. The synaptosome in turn can be further separated into four fractions: the cytoplasm originally present when the synaptosome was formed; mitochondria; synaptic vesicles; and the outer membrane of the nerve terminal, usually obtained with some adhering postsynaptic membrane.

Synaptic membranes contain a number of proteins that differ from those found in mitochondrial membranes. The lipids are characteristically polar, with a high ganglioside content. Enzymes present in the membranes of at least some synaptosomes include cholinesterase and ATP-ase.

The synaptosomal cytoplasm contains a full array of glycolytic enzymes. Lactic dehydrogenase is considered a characteristic enzyme, as is glutamic decarboxylase. Other enzymes of transmitter synthesis, such as tyrosine hydroxylase (Chapter 8), are also present. The few mitochondria present in each synaptosome have not been found to differ substantially from the mitochondria of the perikaryon. Some synaptic vesicles contain dopamine beta hydroxylase, an enzyme that converts dopamine to norepinephrine (Chapter 8). They also contain transmitters stored in stable form. It is believed that there is only one species of transmitter in any one synaptosome.

Regional Distribution

Some of the chemical differentiation that occurs in differing brain regions is obvious from the preceeding outline of morphology and chemistry. White matter, largely composed of myelinated fibers, will have a gross chemical composition characteristic of myelin, while the cerebral cortex, with a high content of perikarya, will have a predictably different array of chemical entities. More detailed examination shows that there are differences between various neuron-rich areas, presumably related to their specialized functions.

The regional localization of transmitter substances is presently under intense investigation. It is clear that most of the brain serotonin (Chapter 8) is found in axon terminals originating from perikarya located in the midbrain raphe nuclei. Terminal branches of their axons project to the globus pallidus, putamen, caudate nucleus, thalamus, and hypothalamus. Perikarya whose axon terminals contain dopamine are also found in large numbers in midbrain nuclei, but their axons project largely to the limbic system, caudate nucleus, and putamen, and not in appreciable numbers to the globus pallidus. Perikarya whose axon terminal contain norepinephrine are localized in large numbers in the medulla and pontine nuclei, and they have axons that project to the hypothalamus, thalamus, and limbic system. Substantial quantities of each of the transmitter amines are found in the hypothalamus and lesser amounts occur in the thalamus. The perikarya of each of these neuronal types contain the respective amine, but in lower concentrations than the terminals.

The dopamine-producing neurons which originate in the substantia nigra of the midbrain and terminate in the caudate (a part of the corpus striatum) are designated as a nigrostriatal system. Other dopamine systems have been identified; for example there is a short path from the tuberal nuclei of the hypothalamus to the pituitary.

The enzymes of transmitter synthesis also show a regional localization. For example, the enzyme tryosine hydroxylase, important in the synthesis of dopamine and norepinephrine (Chapter 8), is 50 times as active in the caudate as in the pons. Choline acetylase, which synthesizes acetyl choline, is five times as active in the caudate as in the cortex of a rabbit brain. Monoamine oxidase exists at the same level of activity in the cortex, caudate, thalamus, and medulla of a rabbit brain.

Gamma aminobutyric acid transaminase, which regulates the level of the inhibitory transmitter gamma aminobutryic acid (Chapter 8), has high activity in the basal ganglia, hypothalamus, and cerebral and cerebellar cortex.

More specific localizations have been studied by means of histochemical techniques. Succinic dehydrogenase (SDH) and cytochrome oxidase (CYO), enzymes in the oxidative phosphorylation pathway, are localized in mitochondria, while lactic dehydrogenase (LDH), an enzyme of glycolysis, is principally found "free" in ctyoplasm. In the supraoptic nucleus of the hypothalamus LDH predominates; in the anterior medial thalamus LDH is lower than the mitochondrial enzymes; in the ventro-lateral thalamus CYO is lower than SDH or LDH; and in the locus caeruleus SDH is lower than the others.

This has been a brief survey of chemical localization in the brain. As is the case with structural anatomy, the subject is far too complex to be treated in detail here. What has been presented is intended as an introduction to the diversity of chemical function at the regional, cellular, and intracellular level. Explanations of behavioral function are not yet known for all of the observed chemical differences, but it will be clear from succeeding chapters that at least such details, and probably studies at other levels of organization, will be needed to approach an understanding of the complexity of brain function.

The preceding outline has purposefully omitted any discussion of the chemical distinctions between neurons and glia, since progress in this area is just beginning. As an example of what might be expected the activity of the enzyme carbonic anhydrase is instructive. This enzyme catalyzes the reaction between water and carbon dioxide to form carbonic acid. It is important in the internal respiration of cells, and also as a source of hydrogen ion (from the carbonic acid) for exchange with cations. Carbonic anhydrase activity is 50 times greater in glia than in neurons. It has been suggested that one function of glial cells might be to take up, and temporarily store, potassium released by neuronal activity. Thus the functional activity of neurons might be directly and instantaneously dependent upon the metabolic activity of neighboring glia cells.

3

Developmental Neurochemistry

THE ELECTROENCEPHALOGRAM OF a premature infant of about 6 months gestational age shows only the barest traces of the patterns that characterize the normal adult. Premature infants of 7 and 8 months gestational age have EEGs with a little more organization. The full-term infant has a more developed EEG pattern, but it is not until 12 months postnatal that an alpha rhythm is clearly present.

The morphological changes that underlie this manifestation of brain function begin with a period of nerve cell division that approaches completion during the 7th embryonic month. From then until birth there is a growth in size of neurons, partly due to the emergence of axons and dendrites. Along with continued growth, myelination begins at about 4 months postnatal and continues thereafter, although growth of neurons almost stops. Division of glial cells apparently continues for the first year of life.

Parallel changes occur in rats, with the time for completion of cell division lasting until birth, growth of axons and dendrites

39

to 10 days postnatal, and rapid myelination occurring between 10 and 20 days postnatal.

Specific details of cell growth are available from experimental studies with rats. In the cerebral cortex the relative proportion of glia to neurons increases throughout life. The packing density of neurons, defined as the number contained in each cubic millimeter of tissue, decreases from about 1.5 million at 10 days to 900,000 at 100 days, in area 2 of the rat cortex (area 2 is a sensory area). The decrease in packing density is partly the result of an increase in brain size; since the number of neurons does not increase after birth, the number per unit volume must decrease as the brain grows. Part of the increased brain size is due to the growth of dendrites and axons. The number of synaptic junctions in the molecular layer of the cerebral cortex increases from 150 million per cubic millimeter at 12 days to 1.5 billion at 26 days. There are therfore about 1,500 synapses on the average neuron, if these separate measurements may be combined. Similar changes occur in other brain regions, although not necessarily at the same time. For example, in the cerebellar cortex of the rat synaptic development begins earlier, at 4 days postnatal, and reaches a maximum at 21 days. Neurochemical development is only roughly predictable from the cytological changes.

Chemical changes in the human brain are known to occur throughout fetal development. During the first 7 months of fetal life, when the principal growth process is the multiplication of neurons, the lipid composition of the brain is relatively constant. At 2 months gestational age cholesterol comprises about 2½ %of the weight of brain solids. At the same time glycolysis becomes operative in the fetal brain. At 10 weeks cholinesterase activity appears in the spinal cord, and at this time lower limb movements become possible. At 3 months there is a small but measurable amount of DNA in the brain. Oxidative metabolism first appears at this time. At 4 to 5 months myelination of the sensory fiber tracts of the spinal cord is in evidence. The following month demosterol, a metabolic precursor in the pathway of cholesterol synthesis, accounts for almost 6% of the total sterols.

Axonal and dendritic growth during the 8th and 9th fetal months results in an increase in ganglioside concentration. At birth the brain gangliosides occur in higher concentration than the cerebrosides. Cholesterol has accumulated to the extent of 5% of the total brain solids, but the fraction of sterols represented by desmosterol has fallen to less than 2%. At birth there are about 700 milligrams of DNA and about 930 milligrams of RNA.

The total weight of the brain, about 250 grams at birth, increases in males up to about age 35 and decreases in later life. This pattern of development is also true for many lipids of the human brain. The ages at which some classes of lipids reach their highest concentrations are listed in Table 3-1. It can be seen from

Table 3-1

CHANGES IN LIPID CONCENTRATION WITH AGE*

Lipid Class	Age of Maximum Concentration
Sulfatide	40 Years
Sphingomyelin	38 years
Cerebroside	21 years
Cholesterol	33 years
Phosphatidalethanolamine	30 years
Phosphatidylethanolamine	30 years
Phosphatidylserine	33 years
Phosphatidylcholine	33 years
Ganglioside	8 months
Cardiolipin	2 years
Phosphatidic acid	Increases throughout life

*Concentration in human brain.

this table that of the lipids characteristic of myelin, cerebroside concentration peaks earliest at 21 years and sulfatide latest at 40 years. The scale of these changes can be appreciated from the following. In each 100 grams of brain there are 2.65 millimoles of cerebroside and 0.67 millimole of sulfatide at age 21. (The term "millimole" is used because it relates directly to the number of molecules of a given substance and thus allows direct comparison between substances of differing molecular weight.) By age 40 there are 1.88 millimoles of cerebroside and 0.78 millimole of sulfatide. Although sulfatides are synthesized from cerebrosides by adding a sulfate group, it is not possible to ascertain from such data alone whether the 0.11 milimole of new sulfatide arose directly, molecule for molecule, from any part of the 0.77 millimole of cerebroside that was lost over this time period.

The changes in myelin with age are more complex, however. Any single molecule of cerebroside or sulfatide contains 1
molecule of a fatty acid. All lipids are made up of classes of compounds, such as cerebrosides, whose members differ from one
another in the kind of fatty acid occurring in each molecule.
There are at least 28 different fatty acids found in cerebrosides.
The same 28 are found in sulfatides. In some instances, such as
that of lignoceric acid, a saturated fatty acid with 24 carbon
atoms, the relative proportion of lignoceryl cerebroside decreases to the same extent as that of lignoceryl sulfatide from age
21 to age 40. In another case, that of stearic acid (an 18 carbon saturated fatty acid), the relative proportion increases in cerebrosides but is unchanged in sulfatides. Thus brain lipids change
continuously with age, not only with respect to the relative proportions of the classes of lipids, but also with respect to the individual members of each class.

The changes, which are so complex as to defy ready gen-
eralization even during the mature years of relatively stable brain
chemistry, are even more complex during the early years of rapid
deposition of myelin. Thus, the lignoceric acid content of myelin
cerebrosides is the same at 10 months and 55 years, from which it
may be inferred that lignoceryl cerebrosides have attained the
"adult pattern" by 10 months. Lignoceryl sulfatides, however, are
more abundant at 10 months than at 55 years, raising the question
as to whether their disappearance with age has any functional
significance.

The decrease in lignoceric acid in sulfatides over the period
10 months to 55 years is exactly balanced by the increase in nervonic acid, a substance which differs from lignoceric acid only in
that there is a double bond (unsaturation) between the 15th and
16th carbon atoms. Despite the similarity, however, lignoceric
acid is not directly converted to nervonic acid. Biologically, lignoceric acid is synthesized by elongation of stearic acid, and
nervonic acid by elongation of oleic acid, which is obtained from
stearic acid by enzyme systems capable of introducing unsaturation. Thus the conversion of lignoceryl to nervonyl sulfatides
during the maturing process probably requires removal of lignoceric acid and incorporation of newly synthesized nervonic acid,
while the remainder of the sulfatide molecule remains locked in

place in the myelin structure. The functional significance of such detailed changes is not presently understood.

Nervonic acid also increases in myelin cerebrosides over the period 10 months to 55 years, but, since lignoceric acid remains unchanged, it is likely that the increase is due either to partial replacement of several of the other fatty acids or to total synthesis and deposition of nervonyl cerebrosides. In either case this detailed example points to the neurochemical independence of these closely related lipid classes during development.

The data cited above were obtained by isolation of myelin from the brain and analysis of its constituents. The techniques of isolation produce at least two myelins, a "heavy" and a "light" fraction. There may be others. An indication that chemical changes may differ among myelin fractions is suggested by the following. Since cerebrosides and sulfatides are widely believed to be located largely, if not exclusively, in myelin, analysis of these lipids extracted directly from the whole brain, without prior isolation of myelin, should give approximately the same results as are obtained when these substances are separated from the myelin fraction. From 6 months to 2 years of age both cerebrosides and sulfatides double their concentration in the whole brain. At the same time cerebronic acid (hydroxylignoceric acid—the 24-carbon saturated fatty acid with a hydroxyl group substituted for one of its hydrogens at a carbon atom) decreases in cerebrosides but increases sharply in sulfatides. In contrast, lignoceric acid increases sharply and stearic acid decreases sharply in each of these lipid classes during the same time period. Looking in more detail at lignoceric acid in the whole brain, the proportion found in cerebrosides at 55 years is only one-half of that found at 1 year. It was noted above that the lignoceric acid of myelin cerebrosides was unchanged over the period 10 months of 55 years. Three explanations are possible. These data, obtained by different laboratories, may be due to differences in technique or available samples; the supposition that cerebrosides are located almost exclusively in myelin may be wrong; there may be another myelin fraction, perhaps "very light," which is not obtained by the usual fractionation procedures, whose cerebroside and sulfatide composition differs appreciably from that of the myelin already studied.

In any case the data already discussed indicate clearly that minute details of myelin composition are subject to change throughout growth and development of the brain. If the function of myelin were simply to provide electrical insulation for the nerve fibers, such changes would be superfluous. It is unlikely that the changes in fatty acid composition of cerebrosides and sulfatides are due to changes in the overall chemical environment, even though it is known that diet does affect the brain's chemistry (Chapter 4), since the reported changes are specific and different for each of these two lipid classes. It is more likely that there are chemically different myelins, subserving different functions, and that their chemical composition is subject to change as different functional requirements arise during development.

Other myelin lipids also show changes in fatty acid composition during development. Thus stearic acid, the major component fatty acid of sphingomyelins at 10 months of age, decreases by half at 55 years, while nervonic acid undergoes a fourfold increase to become a major fatty acid. Phosphatidal serine is a lipid class present in myelin, whose individual members are distinguished by the different kinds of fatty aldehydes that can be obtained from the parent compound (see Figure 3-1). Palmitoyl

$$CH_3-(CH_2)_{14}-\underset{H}{C}=O$$

Palmitoyl aldehyde

$$CH_3-(CH_2)_{16}-\underset{H}{C}=O$$

Stearoyl aldehyde

$$CH_3-(CH_2)_7-CH=CH-(CH_2)_7-\underset{H}{C}=O$$

Oleyl aldehyde

Figure 3-1. Some fatty aldehydes found in brain lipids.

aldehyde, stearyl aldehyde, and oleyl aldehyde are major components at 10 months. The first two are decreased by one-third at age 55, while oleyl aldehyde almost doubles. The pattern is quite similar for phosphatidal ethanolamine, another lipid class present in myelin. Proteins in myelin also change with age with a sizable increase in basic amino acid content. However, the relative proportion of protein to lipid remains constant.

The marked contrast in rate of accumulation between gangliosides and the myelin lipids (Table 3-1) is accounted for by the underlying morphological changes, for gangliosides are present in membranes of perikarya, microsomes, and nerve endings. Before axons can myelinate they must first grow, branch, and form terminals. Hence an increase in gangliosides precedes an increase in myelin lipids. The concentration of gangliosides decreases because more brain volume is occupied by myelinated fibers, and less by terminals, as development proceeds.

Cardiolipin, a lipid found almost entirely in mitochondria, reaches its highest concentration at 2 years (Table 3-1). Phosphatidic acid, which is an intermediate in the synthesis of several phospholipids including cardiolipin, continues to increase in concentration throughout life. No functional relationships for these age-dependent changes are known at the present time.

Other neuronal phospholipids also increase in concentration continuously until about age 30. Multiplication of neurons, as indicated previously, ends at about 7 months gestational age, but an increase in the numbers of neuroglia continues, as evidenced by a continued increase in the DNA content of the whole brain from 700 milligrams at birth to 900 milligrams at 6 months and a final value of 1,000 milligrams by 12 to 15 months. The ratio of RNA to DNA, indicative of growth in size of the average neuron, is 1.3 at 4 days postnatal, 1.7 by 1 year, and 2.6 in the adult. The continued increase in phospholipid concentration is therefore consistent with an increase in average neuronal size well into adult life.

Cellular growth is closely associated with increases in enzymes and other proteins. The cytochromes are iron-containing enzymes. Ferritin is an iron-storage protein. It is known that the total iron content of the brain exists largely in the form of ferritin, with smaller amounts present in the cytochromes, in heme (the pigment of hemoglobin), and as inorganic iron. In the brains of rats and rabbits iron is very labile; injection of lysergic acid diethylamide (LSD) was followed 15 minutes later by a reduction in brain iron. Even so, it has been possible to relate the iron content of the human brain to age. The cerebrum of the human fetus shows an increase in nonheme iron starting with the third month of fetal life and continuing until birth. During childhood and adolescence the iron content of the globus pallidus increases greatly and becomes constant at about 30 years. A smaller increase occurs in the thalamus from birth until age 30, after which there is a decrease. Peak levels are not attained in the putamen and red nucleus until ages 50 to 60.

More detailed information about patterns of protein and enzyme development comes from experimentally controlled studies in rats, rabbits, and other animals. The S-100 protein, specific to the brain (Chapter 2), is almost absent at birth in rats, appears in measurable quantities at 12 to 15 days, and increases about twentyfold in concentration by 60 to 80 days, after which time it is constant. In humans there is an increase in S-100 protein in many, but not all, brain regions from about 16 years of age on, throughout life.

Proteins are synthesized from uncombined amino acids present in the cell cytoplasm. Thus the cytoplasmic amino acid content has some relation to the extent of protein synthesis. Table 3-2

Table 3-2

CHANGES IN AMINO ACID CONCENTRATION WITH AGE*

Amino Acid	Direction of Change
Aspartic acid	Increases
Glutamic acid	Increases
Gamma amino butyric acid	Increases
Glutamine	Decreases
Threonine	Decreases
Proline	Decreases
Glycine	Decreases

*Concentration in the adult rabbit brain compared with concentration in the newborn brain.

lists those amino acids whose concentration in newborn and adult rabbit brains either increases or decreases. All others studied did not change significantly.

The general pattern of appearance of enzymes coincides with the stage of morphological development. The first enzymes

Table 3-3

TIME OF DEVELOPMENT OF SOME ENZYMES
OF THE RAT BRAIN

Enzyme	Age of first appearance	Age of maximum rate of increase
Glucose-6-phosphate dehydrogenase	Constant activity from birth	
Glyceraldehyde phosphate dehydrogenase		5 to 10 days
Esterases	20 days	
Lactic dehydrogenase (LDH-E)		50 days
ATPase	10 days	
Malic dehydrogenase	10 days	
Succinic dehydrogenase		6 to 9 days
Cytochrome oxidase	10 days	
Carbonic anhydrase		20 to 60 days
Gamma amino butyrate transaminase		12 to 26 days

to appear are those required for synthesis of structural components, followed next by the enzymes related to cell differentiation, and finally by those enzymes related to neuronal function. Table 3-3 lists the time of maximum increase of some enzymes of the rat brain.

A "critical period" in development of the rat brain cerebrum has been assigned to the 10- to 14-day postnatal interval. Total brain protein is unchanged from birth until the 10th postnatal day, when a rapid increase in synthesis, lasting about 15 days, is initiated. The 10- to 14-day interval marks the period of greatest morphological change. Purkinje cells of the cerebellar cortex develop their extensive dendritic arborizations; several cerebellar cell types appear or differentiate; myelination, almost non-existent at the 9th day, is extensive at the 14th day. An adult EEG pattern appears at this time.

Just prior to the onset of the critical period there are significant increases in aldolase (an enzyme of the glycolytic sequence) and succinic dehydrogenase (SDH) activity. During the 10- to 14-day period gamma amino butyric acid transaminase (GABA-transaminase) becomes elevated. The latter two enzymes are concerned with the regulation of GABA, a substance which serves both as a transmitter (Chapter 8) and a component of the GABA shunt (Chapter 2). It would seem, then, that during the critical period two pathways of glucose metabolism become more available: glycolysis, which supplies some energy independent of the tricarboxylic acid cycle; and the GABA shunt, which is a variant of a step in the cycle that occurs only in the brain. Another pathway of glucose oxidative metabolism to carbon dioxide, involving intermediate production of pentoses (five carbon sugars found in nucleotides, RNA, and DNA), requires the enzyme glucose -6- phosphate-dehydrogenase, which is relatively constant in activity from birth throughout adult life.

The increased availability of the glycolytic pathway, implied by the increase in aldolase activity, is dependent upon other enzymes as well. One of these, lactic dehydrogenase (LDH), exists as a mixture of five isoenzymes. There are two different polypeptides found in LDH. The functional enzyme is composed of four polypeptide units which may be assembled from any of the five permutations of the two forms. Three of these combinations change during development. The LDH isoenzymes that function best in anaerobic glycolysis (where oxygen supply to the tissue is limited and a large amount of lactic acid is accumulated) decrease in activity from birth on. The LDH isoenzyme that functions best when aerobic glycolysis is called for (lactic acid is removed from the tissue for further metabolism elsewhere)is not present at all at birth but increases thereafter so that by 50 days it constitutes 35% of all the LDH isoenzymes. Thus the brain switches from anaerobic glycolysis, characteristic of the fetal state, to the capacity for aerobic glycolysis soon after birth.

With the onset of functional activity the enzymes that regulate transmitter concentration become more active. Table 3-4 lists the activity of some of these enzymes in the adult rabbit brain relative to that in a brain 3 days old. The ratios are calculated for a constant number of cells (actually, for DNA, which is proportional to the number of cells). The greatest increase in 5-hydroxytryptophan decarboxylase, an enzyme that produces serotonin, occurs in the caudate nucleus. The existence of fiber tracts leading from the serotonin-containing neurons of the midbrain raphe nuclei to the caudate has already been mentioned. The data of Table 3-4 indicate that such pathways become functional as development proceeds. The periods between 12 and 15 days and between 19 and 32 days mark the greatest rate of increase of 5-

Table 3-4

DEVELOPMENTAL CHANGE* OF
RABBIT BRAIN ENZYMES

Enzyme	Brain Region			
	Cortex	Caudate	Thalamus	Medulla
Choline acetylase	12	12	4	3
Choline esterase	9	8	2.5	1
5-hydroxy-tryptophan decarboxylase	9	14	5	2.5
Monoamine oxidase	3	3	.9	1

*The ratio of enzyme activity at maturity to that of three days. In each case the activity is corrected for the content of DNA per gram wet weight of brain tissue and thus represents activity referred to a constant number of cells.

hydroxytryptophan decarboxylase, referred to DNA content.

Along with the rapid and extensive neurochemical changes during early development there are changes in the systems controlling the flow of nutrients through the brain. The blood-brain barriers (Chapter 2) are not nearly as restrictive in the newborn as in the mature animal. Cerebrospinal fluid is first observed in rats 6 days prior to birth. The adult characteristics of cerebrospinal fluid formation, which include active transport of anions and cations across the choroid plexus, is achieved by the 9th postnatal day.

Surveying some of the available information, it is apparent that the chemical structure of the brain is in continuous flux. Although the most obvious changes occur early in development, associated with morphological differentiation and growth, there are a host of subtle alterations in the fine chemical structure of cellular organelles that become evident at various periods. Some of these continue throughout life. The possibility that some of the chemical changes are governed not only by genetic information but also by specific components of the diet will be examined in the next chapter.

4

Malnutrition and Brain Development

RETARDED PHYSICAL GROWTH and development of young children occurs in almost all members of low-income groups in the less industrialized countries. The judgment that growth is retarded is made by comparison with the growth of children of the high-income families in the same countries. Comparisons of the growth of children in widely differing economic groups in the industrialized nations lead to the same conclusions. Although malnutrition has been identified as the principal cause of retarded growth, the causes of malnutrition are varied, including inadequate food supplies, poor dietary practices, and the prevalence of infectious disease. With respect to dietary insufficiency, it is known that a diet low in both protein and caloric content is particularly damaging.

Apathy, low motivation and initiative, poor performance in a variety of intelligence tests, abnormal EEGs, and decreased brain size are prevalent among children who have experienced malnutrition in the first 2 years of life, even if subsequent to that time they received adequate nutrition for up to 10 years. It is also observed that these permanent alterations are more severe, and occur in larger numbers of children, in direct relation to the degree of overlap between the period of malnutrition and the time at which brain growth is normally maximum. Many investigators have argued that malnutrition may not be causal to the observed behavior since such children come from a deprived social mileau. However, the evidence from studies with experimental animals showing a direct effect of malnutrition on neurochemical development, coupled with similar but less frequent neurochemical observations of malnourished humans, strongly supports the conclusion that, to some extent at least, malnutrition in early infancy contributes to irreversible loss of the opportunity for that degree of brain development needed for "normal" intellectual and emotional performance.

The data relating malnutrition to human brain growth are not very extensive. What is known may be summarized as follows. Human infants who died of malnutrition during their first year of life had a lesser brain weight than adequately nourished infants who died of other causes in the same geographical regions. Not only the total weight, but the proportional weight of brain solids, measured after removal of tissue water, was also lower. The total DNA, and therefore the total number of cells, was also decreased in the malnourished infants. In large part the low level of DNA is caused by a decrease in the number of neuroglia, which normally continue to increase after birth. However, some data indicate that a total DNA content of less than half of the expected value occurs at 3 to 6 months of age. This indicates that the number of neurons is also below normal in some instances. RNA and protein are also below normal. Reduction in neuroglia has important consequences, for myelin is produced by the oligodendroglia. Total cholesterol, a myelin component, and phosphatides are also decreased at the same time. Although the lipid data indicate a decrease in the total amount of myelin present, the concentration of lipid in a specified volume of brain is not appreciably affected. It is concluded from these observations that the thickness of existing myelin is unchanged. Thus the already existing oligodendroglia have functioned normally to produce myelin. However, either the number or length of myelinated axons is reduced because of an insufficiency of new oligodendroglia. Furthermore, the average size of a neuron, including perikaryon, dendrites, and axon, is reduced. Gangliosides, whose presence is indicative of synaptic endings, also occur in lower concentrations. It is apparent from this that the growth of myelinated interconnections between neurons is impaired by severe malnutrition occurring up to the first 2 years of life. This limited time, during which an event must happen or else the opportunity for it to occur is forever lost, is called a "critical period." Studies of the effects of maternal malnutrition show that the stillborn fetus has a decreased number of brain cells.

Controlled studies of undernutrition in experimental animals, coupled with the well-established correlations between the normal neurochemical structure of human and other species of mammalian brain, give additional insight into the probable effects of malnutrition on the chemical structure of the human brain.

As discussed in Chapter 2, the characteristic lipids of myelin are cholesterol, cerebrosides, sphingomyelin, and phosphatidalethanolamine. If myelination is diminished as a result of malnutrition it would be expected that the total amount of each of these lipids present in the brain would be decreased in proportion to its fractional amount of the total myelin lipids. An experimental study with pigs, severely undernourished from the age of 2 weeks to 1 year, produced a surprising result. A 29% reduction in DNA occurred, when compared with well-nourished controls, as expected from many other studies. A 34% decrease in nonmyelin lipids also occurred. However, of the myelin lipids, the reduction in cerebrosides was 36%, in cholesterol 21%, while no reduction at all occurred in sphingomyelin or phosphatidalserine. The difference in the extent of cerebroside and cholesterol deficiencies could be interpreted to mean that a substantial amount of cholesterol is present in nonmyelinated structures, whereas the cerebroside reduction was more extensive since all of it was present in myelin. But the lack of any significant change in the other two components of myelin is unexplained by such reasoning. The possible explanations include the following: partial myelination, utilizing sphingomyelin and phosphatidalserine, can occur in the absence of oligodendroglia; more than one kind of oligodendroglia exists, and only those producing a cholesterol-cerebroside myelin are affected by undernutrition; undernutrition leads to a large deficiency in the enzymes or the precursors of cholesterol and cerebroside synthesis, while phosphatidalserine and sphingomyelin synthesis is unaffected and therefore favored. In any case it is clear that all of these explanations assume not only a decrease in the amount of myelin formed but also a simultaneous production of an atypical myelin.

The experiment with the undernourished pigs was continued by supplying some of them with adequate nutrition for the next 2½ years. The nonmyelin lipids returned to normal, the DNA deficit was reduced from the 29% at 1 year to 14%, the cholesterol deficit was reduced from 21% to 13%, and the cerebroside deficit was reduced from 36% to 14%. The major conclusion from these experiments is that renutrition could not completely reverse the damage and that a gross deficiency remained in cell number and in cerebrosides and cholesterol. The relative gain in these lipids seemed to correlate well with a gain in cell number, as evidenced by the increase in DNA. However, the evidence for the presence of an atypical myelin remains.

Undernutrition in rats prior to weaning has been produced by adding to the normal litter of 10 an additional 6 to 10 animals taken from other litters. The smaller litters are then regarded as an overnourished group. Studies in rats undernourished during the first 3 weeks of life by this technique have produced a similar picture, with some added details. Sulfatides are incorporated into myelin lipids at a reduced rate, and the enzyme responsible for their formation by addition of a sulfate group to cerebrosides is also present in reduced quantity. This indirectly supports the third explanation listed above for the differential effects of undernutrition on pig brain cerebrosides and sphingomyelin, since it shows that a specific enzyme deficiency can occur.

Not only lipid but also proteolipid protein of myelin is reduced as a result of undernutrition of rats during the preweaning period. Restoration of adequate nutrition after the 21st day resulted in variable data; some rats appeared to regain the missing proteolipids and cerebrosides, while others were permanently deficient. Since brains taken from control rats at specific time points also contained widely varying amounts of myelin lipids it appears that there may be an interplay of other factors with the experimentally produced undernutrition. The experimental study of nutrition-dependent brain growth has only recently begun in a few laboratories; variable data at this stage are to be expected.

If reproducible changes in brain chemistry are hard to obtain as a consequence of undernutrition during the critical early phase of neuronal increase in size and glial cell multiplication, it would seem inordinately harder to link later changes in brain chemistry with the quality of the diet. Undernutrition after the critical age does not result in observable deficits in the neurochemical structure of the brain. Does this mean that subsequent brain function is independent of dietary factors?

It is known (Chapter 3) that the fine neurochemical structure of the brain continues to change throughout life, both with respect to the relative proportions of the constituent lipid classes of myelin and also with respect to the detailed fatty acid composition of each class. To date there have been no experiments designed to examine the possibility that such chemical changes correlate with alterations in behavioral performance of experimental animals. However, there are a number of specific nutritional deficiencies of humans which do have strong behavioral correlations. At this point the distinction must be emphasized between the undernourished rats, receiving a balanced but inadequate food supply, and the malnourished patient whose diet, although quantitatively adequate, may be deficient in some particular component.

Such specific deficiencies occur occasionally as a result of insufficient vitamin intake. For example, a diet containing less than 150 micrograms per day of thiamine (Vitamin B_1) may result after only 4 to 5 days in a neurasthenic syndrome, with the major symptoms being lassitude, irritability, and anorexia. If the diet contains 450 micrograms per day, several weeks are required before the syndrome becomes evident. The symptoms usually disappear within 3 to 6 days after returning to a normal diet containing 1 to 2 milligrams of thiamine per day. A more severe consequence results from a dietary insufficiency of thiamine coupled with alcoholism; here the symptoms may progress to include damage to the peripheral nerves and a disordered consciousness usually accompanied by irreversible neuronal damage. At this stage treatment with thiamine may not reverse all the symptoms; the remaining symptom complex is known as the Korsakoff syndrome, characterized by failure of recent memory, confabulation, and disorientation. The usual daily requirement for thiamine is not constant; high carbohydrate diets must be supplemented with increased thiamine intake. It is needed, of course, in all other body tissues as well as the brain. The normal thiamine content of the cerebral cortex may be reduced by half during chronic alcoholism, high fever, or persistent vomiting, all coupled with some degree of undernutrition.

Another example of a well-studied vitamin deficiency, with central nervous system consequences, is that of niacin. A severe lack of this vitamin is associated with pellagra, a nutritional deficiency disease characterized by dermatitis, and in severe cases by extensive hemorrhagic damage to the gastrointestinal tract. Before such symptoms develop, deprivation of niacin leads to mental symptoms that may include some or all of the following: depression, dizziness, apprehension, hallucinations, and disorientation. The symptoms are reversed by niacin. In the continued absence of niacin neuronal damage results.

Vitamin B_{12} deficient diets, clearly associated with pernicious anemia, also lead to neurological damage which may occur independently of the anemia. Loss of myelin, first from peripheral nerves and later from axons in the central nervous system, has been demonstrated to result from B_{12} deficiency at any age. Mental effects associated with the deficiency include: depression, and other changes in affect; hallucinations and paranoid psychosis; confusion, delusion, and poor memory. Impairment of memory is most clearly demonstrated to be associated with B_{12} deficiency; improvement and return to normal occurred within 2 weeks after the start of B_{12} therapy.

Although other examples could be cited, these will suffice to illustrate that the structural integrity of the brain is dependent throughout life on some key nutritional factors. It is obvious that such relationships between the brain and diet are easily demonstrated only when there are severe clinical consequences of a dietary deficiency. Subtler behavioral changes, which could be either advantageous or disadvantageous, conceivably could be associated with the changes known to occur throughout life in the fine details of neurochemical structure, such as in the fatty acid composition of cerebrosides. The impetus to look for such associations is apparently still some distance in the future.

At the beginning of this chapter it was mentioned that the causal relationship between childhood undernutrition and impaired brain function in later life has been questioned on the grounds that such children come from a deprived social mileau which might have produced the observed functional deficits. Although it is clear from all of the foregoing that undernutrition during the critical period leads to reduced brain growth which must be expressed in some way as a functional deficit, there is some evidence from studies with rats to show that brain structure and growth are also related to the social environment.

The experimental technique employed to investigate this question is to raise groups of rats in either an "enriched" or a "restricted" environment. Enrichment was achieved by frequent handling and by larger cages with more objects to explore. Rats handled prior to weaning performed better at learning tasks than did the unhandled controls. They also had increased weight of the cerebral cortex and increased content of total protein and of cholinesterase of the brain. An increased glial content was apparently associated with earlier myelination. It has also been observed that the synaptic junction area is increased with the enriched environment.

It thus appears that growth and development of the brain is dependent not only upon adequate nutrition, which provides the material basis for neuronal structure, but also upon adequate information input which possibly provides the stimulus for effective utilization of the chemical substrates.

5

Inborn Chemical Abnormalities

THERE ARE A number of genetically transmitted diseases which are characterized as "metabolic errors." In each case a defect in a gene leads to failure to synthesize a particular enzyme. The lack of the enzyme causes an excessive accumulation of the substance on which it would normally act. There are more than 40 metabolic errors already described where the consequences of the error include brain damage in addition to severe disturbances of other organs.

Notwithstanding the apparent inexorability of the process—a damaged gene linked to a missing enzyme linked in turn to an excessive quantity of metabolite—the cerebral symptoms of the disease may vary greatly among those affected, even in the case of identical twins.

Variations in symptoms of brain damage may relate to the precise age at which the deficiency becomes critical or to other presently unknown environmental factors. There is a formal correspondence between the variable symptoms of undernutrition and the genetic metabolic diseases. The stage of brain development during which undernutrition is incurred determines the subsequent course of neurological damage. Similarly, the enzyme in question may not participate in neurological processes until a required level of maturation is achieved. At that time its lack will be critical to the further course of developmental chemistry. Enzyme deficits may occur at several locations in a reaction sequence leading to synthesis or catabolism of a particular substance; each specific enzyme deficit blocks further metabolism, leading to excessive accumulation of one particular metabolite in the biochemical chain. Each block, associated in this manner with a specific substance, leads to a separate identifiable genetic disease. In formal terms, if in the sequence A→B→C→D each step requires a unique enzyme, the genetic damage may lead to an A- or B- or C-abundant disease. The diseases are generally named according to the characteristic compound in the sequence.

Sphingolipidoses

As the name implies, these are metabolic diseases resulting from errors of sphingolipid metabolism. The particular class of compound involved ranges from sphingomyelin and cerebrosides to a variety of gangliosides (see Chapter 2).

Niemann-Pick Disease

This term actually denotes a group of distinct diseases. The infantile form is the most prevalent. It occurs predominantly among Jews. The central nervous system (CNS) symptoms, which may become evident at any time up to 1 year of age, include slow psychomotor development accompanied by feeding difficulty and vomiting, ataxia (muscular incoordination), tremor and convulsions. There is extensive involvment of other organs. Death usually occurs by age 3. Very similar symptoms characterize the juvenile form of the disease, where the onset usually occurs between ages 1 to 5. Survival may be extended to adolescence. Some cases are known in which the first symptoms occurred after age 5 and survival was extended into adult life. In some of these cases the CNS symptoms consisted of emotional and thought disturbances together with some movement and speech difficulties.

Visible damage to the brain includes a reduced weight, distended neurons, and some demyelination. All forms of the disease are characterized by an accumulation of sphingomyelin, most typically in the spleen and liver, where a twentyfold increase can occur. In the brain, sphingomyelin accumulates more in gray matter than in white; myelin may have a normal sphingomyelin content. Most of the excess in the brain is located in abnormal membrane-bounded structures in the cytoplasm. Other lipids also accumulate; cholesterol, cerebrosides, and some gangliosides are prominent.

So far as is known, there is only one deficient enzyme in Nieman-Pick's disease. Sphingomyelin is normally cleaved by the enzyme sphingomyelinase to phosphorylcholine and a ceramide. (Figure 5-1). This enzyme has been shown to be either absent or present in reduced quantities in several tissues, including the liver, spleen, leukocytes, and bone marrow cells. It has been possible to diagnose the disease prenatally by demonstrating a deficit of the enzyme in cells obtained from amniotic fluid.

Some cases are known without any CNS involvement, but with an accumulation of sphingomyelin and with the characteristic deficiency of sphingomyelinase. All systemic symptoms are present, including enlarged liver, spleen, and lymph nodes, jaundice, and the characteristic Nieman-Pick cells in many organs. These patients can survive for many years. This form of the disease is genetically distinct from the more prevalent form with CNS symptoms.

The variability in CNS symptoms, as well as the accumulation of excess quantities of other lipids, suggests that the CNS expression of the genetic defect may involve some precisely timed interactions between the normally developing brain and a neurochemical disturbance brought on by the interaction of the enzyme deficiency with some environmental factor. Alternatively, the existence of a genetically distinct variant without CNS effects suggests that the genetic timing of normal brain development may be variable, with only minimal consequences of the enzyme deficiency resulting from some favorable combinations of time of development with time of deficiency. Whether these or other conjectures ultimately turn out to be accurate, it is clear that even in this relatively simple case of a single enzyme deficiency there is a wide range of CNS damage, varying from

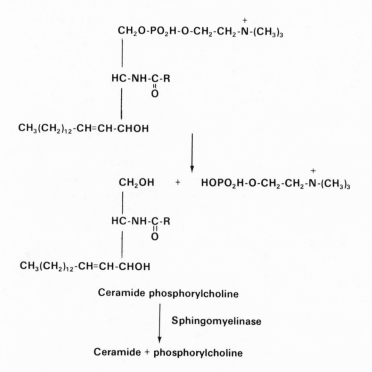

Figure 5-1. The enzymatic block in Nieman-Pick disease.

neurological insufficiency and early death to disturbed emotions in early life.

Metachromatic Leukodystrophy

There are three clinical variations—infantile, juvenile, and adult—known for this disease. They are genetically distinct, with only one variant occurring in a given family. Unlike Nieman-Pick disease there is no ethnic concentration in the cases reported. The infantile form first develops between the 1st and 2nd years of life. Its early stage is characterized by a regression in psychomotor development and by apathy. There is a progressive loss of myelin, leading to spasticity, blindness, and death by age 5.

The onset of the juvenile form is between ages 5 and 15. Intellectual performance is decreased and psychomotor symptoms may appear. Further progression of the disease leads to spasticity and ataxia as the terminal phase is approached. The adult form may become noticeable after adolescence, with behavioral changes predominating. Depression and schizoid behavior may be the initial symptoms. Eventually spasticity occurs. Survival may extend well into middle life.

Loss of myelin from the white matter is extensive, but subcortical association fibers are relatively unaffected. Astrocytes increase in size and number, acting as phagocytes to the damaged myelin. Abnormal granules, found within the white matter, are the most prominant microscopic feature of the disease. The reaction of these granules with a purple dye to produce a yellow-brown color is the basis for the term "metachromatic" in the name of the disease.

Chemically, the disease is characterized by greatly increased quantities of sulfatides and decreased amounts of cerebrosides. These changes are associated with an abnormal myelin. In addition, the metachromatic granules also contain a large amount of sulfatide. In the adult form of the disease white matter sulfatides are double the normal amount, but in the gray matter the increase is fourfold. The increases in sulfatides are due to a deficiency of the enzyme cerebroside sulfatase, which normally converts sulfatide to cerebroside and sulfate (Figure 5-2). There is no striking difference in the extent of the deficiency in the infantile or juvenile forms of the disease compared with the adult form.

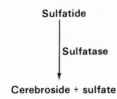

Sulfatide

Sulfatase

Cerebroside + sulfate

Figure 5-2. The enzymatic block in metachromatic leukodystrophy.

Thus, as in the case of Nieman-Pick disease, there are a wide range of symptoms for causes which are presently unknown. A disease which has clear neurological signs in its infant form may, in the adult form, begin with little more than disturbance of affect.

Tay-Sachs Disease

The symptoms of this disease, which are entirely neurological, include muscle weakness by 6 months of age, psychomotor retardation by 1 year, followed by blindness, deafness, and more severe symptoms until death occurs at age 3. Most of the cases known occurred among Jews whose ancestors lived in a small part of Eastern Europe, but there are a few cases among other ethnic groups.

There is extensive swelling of neurons in the brain together with demyelination and an accompanying increase in astrocytes. Neuronal cytoplasm always contains abnormal structures known as membranous cytoplasmic bodies. Although there are no neurological symptoms at birth, morphological changes begin in the fetal brain.

The characteristic chemical substance of Tay-Sachs disease is a monosialoganglioside (Figure 5-3) which increases to several

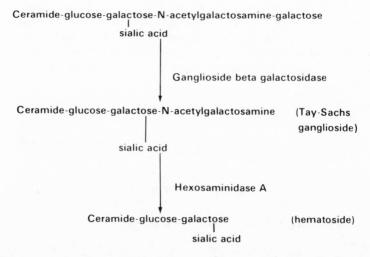

Figure 5-3. Metabolism of a monosialoganglioside. A deficiency of hexosaminidase A leads to an accumulation of the abnormal monosialoganglioside.

hundred times its normal amount, ultimately accounting for 80% to 90% of all the gangliosides. Total ganglioside content is increased to two to three times normal in gray matter. Of the weight of the membranous cytoplasmic bodies 30% is due to gangliosides. The enzyme that is deficient is known as hexosaminidase A. This enzyme is also absent or reduced in blood plasma and leukocytes obtained from patients or their parents. This observation makes genetic counseling possible. Prenatal diagnosis can be made from analysis of amniotic fluid cells.

A juvenile form of the disease has been observed, where the initial symptoms were personality changes followed by progressive psychosis. None of the patients afflicted with this form of the disease was Jewish. The monosialoganglioside accumulation was less extensive than in the infantile form of the disease. Hexosaminidase A was present, but in a reduced quantity.

Diseases of Amino Acid Metabolism

Large excesses of individual amino acids may result from deficiencies of enzymes which are needed for their further metabolism. In those cases where the excess originates in some peripheral organ there is also a large increase in the concentration in the blood plasma, and as a consequence the concentration in the brain is also increased. The symptoms include speech disorders, mental retardation, ataxia, and convulsions. Treatment, if instituted early in infancy, can prevent these symptoms from occurring. In many cases the required treatment is no more than a diet chosen to minimize the particular amino acid.

Phenylketonuria

The biochemical outline of this disease is presented in Figure 5-4. The dietary amino acid phenylalanine is normally metabolized by two pathways. One, common to all amino acids, is the oxidative pathway, leading in this case to phenylpyruvic acid. The other, requiring two enzyme systems, results in the formation of tyrosine. In the absence of one of these enzymes phenylalanine is metabolized solely to phenylpyruvic acid, which is then excreted in the urine in large amounts. (The C=O moiety in phenylpyruvic acid is known as a keto group, hence the name phenylketonuria.)

Mental retardation is an inevitable consequence of untreated

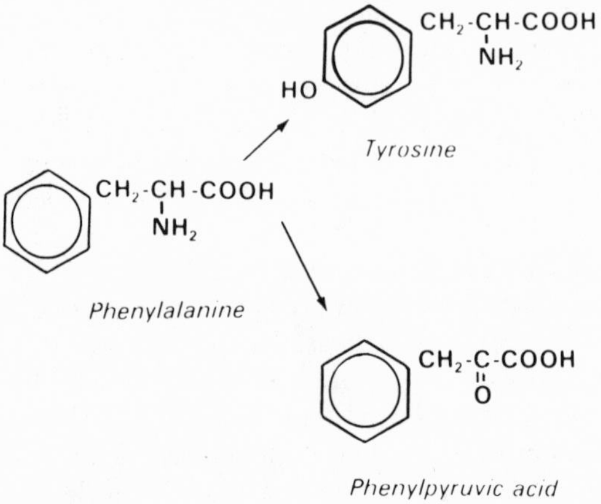

Figure 5-4. Alternate metabolic paths of phenylalanine. Conversion to phenylpyruvic acid is effected by an amino acid oxidase. Conversion to tyrosine requires a pteridine coenzyme and two enzyme systems. One of these is lacking in phenylketonuria.

phenylketonuria. Treatment after 6 months of age will not reverse the damage, but treatment initiated within the first few months of life results in almost normal intellectual development. The treatment consists of a special diet with a carefully regulated quantity of phenylalanine; complete elimination of this amino acid is undesirable since it is essential for many growth processes and cannot be synthesized by the body. The diet is usually maintained up to ages 4 to 10.

The brain of an untreated patient usually weighs less than normal. There is a reduction in the amount of myelin present; however, the myelin composition is apparently normal. It seems certain that the lowered quantity of myelin is due to lack of formation rather than to demyelination.

When infant monkeys were fed large amounts of phenylalanine they subsequently showed impairment of learning. Injections of phenylalanine into rats resulted in a reduced accumulation of many amino acids by the brain because of a competition for transport sites at the blood-brain barrier. The immediate result is an imbalance of amino acids in the brain, leading

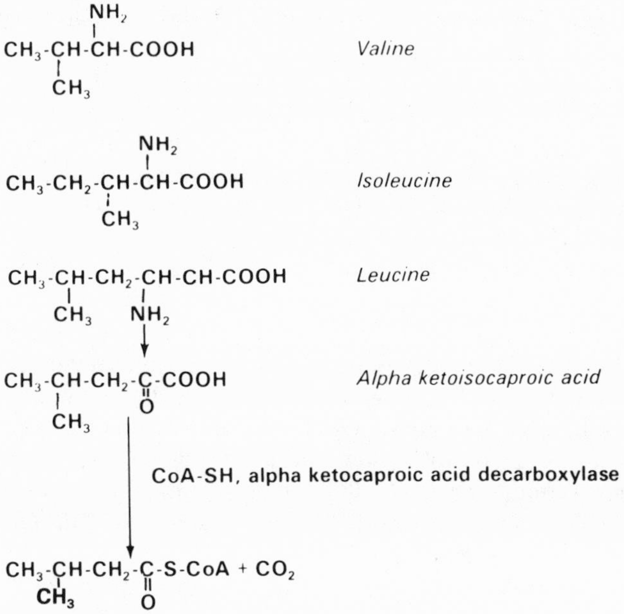

$$CH_3\text{-}CH\text{-}CH\text{-}COOH \qquad \textit{Valine}$$
with NH_2 on the second carbon and CH_3 below

$$CH_3\text{-}CH_2\text{-}CH\text{-}CH\text{-}COOH \qquad \textit{Isoleucine}$$
with NH_2 above and CH_3 below

$$CH_3\text{-}CH\text{-}CH_2\text{-}CH\text{-}CH\text{-}COOH \qquad \textit{Leucine}$$
with CH_3 and NH_2 below

$$CH_3\text{-}CH\text{-}CH_2\text{-}C\text{-}COOH \qquad \textit{Alpha ketoisocaproic acid}$$
with CH_3 below and O (double bond)

CoA-SH, alpha ketocaproic acid decarboxylase

$$CH_3\text{-}CH\text{-}CH_2\text{-}C\text{-}S\text{-}CoA + CO_2$$
with CH_3 below and O (double bond)

Figure 5-5. The enzymatic block in leucinosis. Valine and isoleucine are decarboxylated by other enzymes.

to impairment of protein synthesis. Thus phenylketonuria produces a deficit of some amino acids in the brain, in much the same manner as does protein undernutrition (Chapter 4). The consequences, in both cases, include permanent mental retardation if the deficit occurs during a critical period of development.

Maple Syrup Urine Disease (Leucinosis)

The strange name of this disease arises from the characteristic odor of urine of affected infants. Untreated cases suffer severe neurological damage, coma, and death within a few months of birth. The nonfatal variants, and those for whom diagnosis and treatment is delayed for more than a few days after birth, have severe mental retardation as well as demyelination.

At the present time it appears that there are several genetic variants, leading to inability to decarboxylate the keto acids

arising from the amino acids leucine, isoleucine, and valine
(Figure 5-5). There is a possibility, however, that a primary genetic deficiency of the enzyme alpha-ketoisocaproic acid decarboxylase subsequently leads to a permanent loss of the activity of the other decarboxylases acting on isoleucine and valine.
Further complicating the genetic interpretations are the observations that the enzyme deficiencies occur to differing degrees in
different tissues obtained from the same patient. In addition, it
has been found that the rapidly fatal form is associated with an almost total enzyme deficiency, whereas the other two variants
have higher enzyme levels. In one of these there is just enough enzyme to provide for the patient's normal requirements except
when he is stressed by some other illness, usually an infection.

The biochemical consequences of the enzyme deficiencies
include an increase in the blood, urine, and tissue concentrations
of the three amino acids and their corresponding keto acids. The
chemical substance responsible for the characteristic urine odor
has not yet been identified.

The neurochemical mechanisms associated with mental retardation in this disease are currently under investigation. It is
known that the alpha keto acids are effective agents for the release of stored insulin. It is also known that a reduction in blood
glucose level is associated with increased levels of the three amino
acids in the blood. Thus the increased release of insulin stimulated by the alpha keto acids would lower the already depleted
blood glucose, with immediate consequences to brain function.
Parenthetically, it should be noted that a disease known as
familial hypoglycemia is brought about by certain dietary proteins as well as leucine, isoleucine, or alpha-ketoisocaproic acid;
the symptoms include abnormalities of the electroencephalogram and convulsions.

The keto acid derived from leucine (alpha-ketoisocaproic
acid), but not those derived from isoleucine or valine, inhibits the
enzyme pyruvic decarboxylase when the source of the enzyme is
either the rat or human brain. Phenylpyruvic acid, present in excess in phenylketonuria (see above), also inhibits pyruvic decarboxylase. This enzyme (also known as pyruvic dehydrogenase) is required for the formation of acetyl coenzyme A, a key
intermediate in many biochemical processes. The effect of alpha-

ketoisocaproic acid thus appears to be twofold; it decreases the glucose available to the brain and lowers the conversion of glucose, through pyruvate, to acetyl coenzyme A. How or whether these effects relate to mental retardation is a matter for future research.

Treatment, diagnosis, and genetic counseling are much the same for leucinosis as for phenylketonuria. Diets with reduced contents of the amino acids are provided during early development, with care to provide at least those amounts needed for normal protein synthesis. There are some reports that the proper balance between each of the three amino acids is also important in treatment. Eventually the synthetic diet can be replaced with a diet of natural proteins carefully chosen to limit the intake of the three amino acids.

Other Disorders

Galactosemia

Galactose is metabolized by the addition of a phosphate group to the carbon atom designated as number 1, followed by a sequence of reactions which isomerizes galactose to glucose (Figure 5-6). The first step is effected by the enzyme galacto-

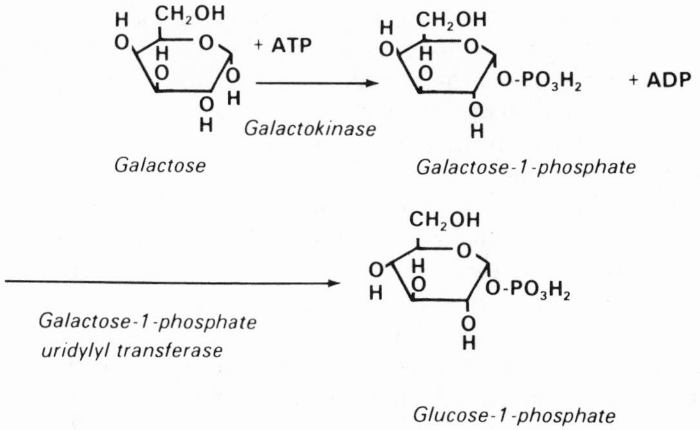

Figure 5-6. Conversion of galactose to glucose-1-phosphate. The transferase enzyme is absent in galactosemia.

kinase. The first reaction in the second sequence requires the enzyme galactose-1-phosphate uridylyl transferase. Two genetic disorders are known, in which either the kinase or the transferase is absent. Galactose and galactitol (the reduction product of galactose) are accumulated with either deficiency; galactose-1-phosphate also accumulates with the transferase deficiency.

Galactose is derived from lactose normally present in milk; hence infants with either form of the disease have elevated blood galactose concentrations. The disease characterized by galactokinase deficiency results in cataracts and no other symptoms. The transferase deficiency produces, in addition to cataracts, enlarged spleen and liver, impaired growth, and mental retardation. Large quantities of amino acids appear in the urine.

This disease is not usually manifested at birth, but it becomes severe when a diet containing lactose is ingested. Jaundice, lethargy, and anorexia are among the first symptoms; a progressively worsening course may lead to early death. Diagnosis can be made by analyzing erythrocytes for the transferase enzyme. Treatment consists in prompt institution of a low galactose diet. Mental retardation is less severe and even absent in a few cases when treatment was begun at birth.

The study of the chemical and physical mechanisms leading to cataract formation in galactosemia has been aided by the observation that when rats are fed a diet containing a large amount of galactose they too develop cataracts. The earliest changes are associated with the enzymatic reduction of galactose to the sugar alcohol, galactitol, in the lens. Galactitol, once formed in the lens, does not diffuse out readily. As its concentration increases there is a compensating flow of water into the lens. (The total concentration of solutes on both sides of a membrane must be the same to maintain osmotic equilibrium.) The total volume of fluid in the lens is therefore increased, causing it to swell. Fibers in the lens rupture, leading to formation of vacuoles which are the earliest sign of the cataract. These changes are soon followed by a loss of amino acids from the lens, as well as by a change in the normal distribution of sodium and potassium in the lens. Both effects are secondary consequences of the initial osmotic changes. The loss of amino acids leads to a decrease in protein synthesis. The increase in galactitol, observed in the lens under carefully controlled conditions, also occurs in the brains of rats fed excess galactose and galactosemic infants who died of the disease. Presumably the secondary osmotic changes demonstrated for the lens also occurred in the brain.

Since galactitol is accumulated both in the kinase and the transferase deficiency and mental retardation only occurs in the latter, it seems clear that the brain can tolerate such changes without undergoing permanent damage. Rather, there may be reversible change in function, as occurs in peripheral nerves of rats fed galactose. In such studies it was found that there was osmotic swelling and that the rate at which the nerve conducted an impulse decreased. However, when galactose was removed from the diet for 2 days all of these changes were reversed.

There is, then, substantial information about changes in brain chemistry which can occur without causing mental retardation. The biochemical effects of galactose-1-phosphate, which accumulates in the transferase deficiency, are presently under intensive study. This substance has been shown to inhibit phosphoglucomutase, an enzyme which switches a phosphate group from the number 1 to the number 6 carbon atom of glucose. Lack of the use of this enzyme would make it impossible to use glucose as an energy source. It has also been suggested that the excess galactose-1-phosphate might combine with protein directly or intefere with RNA metabolism to produce damage to cellular processes.

Lesch-Nyhan Syndrome

This group of symptoms, composed of mental retardation, athetoid movements (an uncontrolled slow writhing and twisting), and self-mutilation, principally by biting, occurs exclusively in males, as a genetic X-linked recessive disease. The first symptoms appear at 6 to 8 months. The ability to sit and hold the head upright is reduced and finally lost entirely. The self-mutilation, which is characteristic of the disease, occurs even though the patients perceive pain acutely and sometimes scream with pain while they bite themselves. They are reported to call for help during periods of self-mutilation. They also engage in aggressive activity against others, limited of course by their lack of muscular control. Other symptoms are related to the fact that uric acid is found in excessive amounts in the blood, urine, and various tissues and organs. The patients may thus suffer from the symptoms of gout.

Although there is a good deal of information relating to the biochemical basis of the disease, it is not yet complete enough to devise a treatment. It is known that there is an overproduction of uric acid. An outline of its biosynthetic pathway is presented in Figure 5-7. The basic structure of uric acid is the purine ring (Figure 2-11). Of the 4 nitrogen atoms in the ring, 2 are derived from glutamine, 1 from aspartic acid, and 1 from glycine. Of the 5

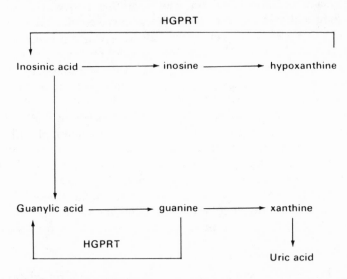

Figure 5-7. The metabolic blocks in Lesch-Nyhan syndrome. Absence of HGPRT leads to an excess conversion of nucleotides to uric acid.

carbon atoms, 2 are derived from glycine, 2 from formate (via folic acid derivatives), and 1 from carbon dioxide. Complete synthesis of the purine rings from these components is referred to as de novo synthesis. The de novo pathway leads directly to the nucleotide, inosinic acid. This compound is the source of the other nucleotides, adenylic and guanylic acids. In addition to the de novo route there is a reutilization step, by which the purines hypoxanthine and guanine are condensed with ribose phosphate (ribose is a sugar with 5 carbon atoms). The enzyme required for this step is called hypoxanthine-guanine phosphoribosyl transferase (HGPRT). It is this enzyme that is absent in the Lesch-Nyhan syndrome.

Excretion of one of the intermediates of purine synthesis, aminoamidazol-4-carboxamide, is increased to 20 times the normal amount in this disease. This observation, coupled with quantitative measurements of the extent of conversion of glycine to uric acid, as well as observations of the rate of conversion of formate to a purine intermediate by cells obtained from Lesch-Nyhan patients, points strongly to the conclusion that the rate of de novo synthesis is excessive in patients suffering from this disease. It seems likely that the lack of the enzyme HGPRT, necessary for reutilization of purines, would be expressed as a failure of feedback inhibition of the de novo synthesis.

How these facts relate to the mental symptoms is not at all clear. There is a variation of the disease in which HGPRT is present at about 5% of normal activity; although overproduction of purines, as well as gout, occurs in these patients, they do not have behavioral or neurological damage. It would seem that at least some of the reutilization pathway is critical for normal brain development and function and that damage is only manifested in its total absence.

Disorders of Vitamin B_{12} Metabolism

In addition to the well-known effects of B_{12} on pernicious anemia, there are several genetic diseases of B_{12} deficiency characterized by mental retardation, cerebellar and spinal cord malfunction, or early death. Vitamin B_{12} is a required component of the human diet. Its entrance into the bloodstream, however, is dependent upon four proteins, each of which may be lacking in a particular genetic disease. The first step after ingestion requires binding to a glycoprotein secreted by the gastric mucosa (the so-called "intrinsic factor"). The B_{12} glycoprotein complex moves to the small intestine, where it attaches to specific receptor sites. The next step is transfer to the bloodstream where the B_{12} link to the glycoprotein is broken and new complexes with two specific proteins are established. Finally, B_{12} is converted to specific coenzymes by reaction with other enzymes.

One of the consequences of ineffective B_{12} utilization is the excretion of large amounts of methylmalonic acid in the urine. This substance, although normally present as a trace metabolite in the body, is an essential link in the metabolism of many substances (Figure 5-8). Its conversion to succinyl coenzyme A is ef-

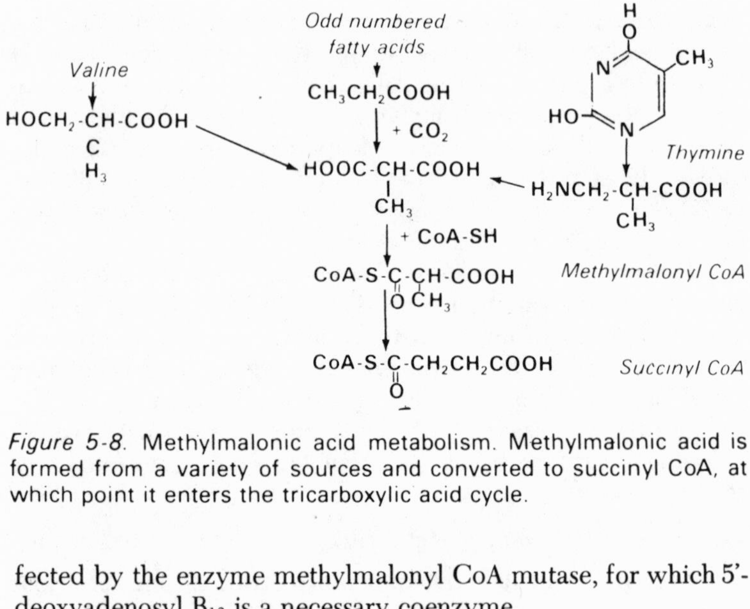

Figure 5-8. Methylmalonic acid metabolism. Methylmalonic acid is formed from a variety of sources and converted to succinyl CoA, at which point it enters the tricarboxylic acid cycle.

fected by the enzyme methylmalonyl CoA mutase, for which 5'-deoxyadenosyl B_{12} is a necessary coenzyme.

In the case of this particular deficiency it has been reported that the retarded development of the central nervous system was reversed with large doses of B_{12}, limited protein ingestion, and treatment of the acidosis produced by the large amount of methylmalonic acid. There are other B_{12} disorders which are not well understood at present. Knowledge of this group of diseases, however, is quite recent and further progress is anticipated by researchers in this field.

6

Chemical Imprinting

It HAS BEEN known for a century that very young birds of certain species will approach and follow the first moving object they encounter. Normally this behavior pattern is expressed as a fixed relation between the young bird and its mother; once established no other object serves as an attractant. However, if the first moving object encountered is another species of bird, a human, or even a mechanical object, the young bird will follow it thereafter, totally disregarding the mother bird. These unique behavior patterns are referred to as imprinting. They can be established only during a limited period during the early life of the bird. For mallard ducklings the critical period occurs during the 5th to the 24th hours after hatching.

The imprinting phenomenon is defined by the brief span of the critical period during which it can be established and by its persistence throughout the life of the animal. Imprinting has been observed in various mammals, ranging from guinea pigs and lambs to zebras. It is believed to be a factor in the poor social adjustment of rhesus monkeys who are reared in isolation during the 3rd to 6th months of life.

Imprinting, although first discovered as a response to a moving object, has recently been observed as a response to other visual stimuli such as flickering lights, and to auditory stimuli as well. Insofar as it is characterized by a critical period in the early life of the animal, it appears to be related to the critical periods of early morphological and neurochemical development which, when interrupted by malnutrition or genetic deficiency diseases, lead to long-term defects in neurological, emotional, or intellectual performance.

The correspondence becomes closer when one considers that neurochemical interventions can disrupt the imprinting process. For example, if an inhibitor of protein synthesis is injected into chicks at times ranging from a few hours to a few days after hatching, it can be demonstrated that maximum impairment of auditory imprinting occurs at 6 hours and of visual imprinting 3 days after hatching. The neurochemical requirements for the imprinting process, although not yet fully explored, are strongly hinted at by these observations. An early experience, central to further development, is rendered permanent by interaction with some neurochemical factors. The analogous effect, in which the presence of a neurochemical factor early in life is central to the determination of some behavior of the adult animal, is the subject of the remainder of this chapter.

A single dose of estrogen (a female sex hormone), given to female rats 4 days after birth, caused profound disruption in the sexual function of the mature animal, including ovarian dysfunction and a complete lack of sexual receptivity. The same hormone, administered at the same age to male rats, similarly had major effects on the adult animal, including total inability to ejaculate, misdirected mounting of females, and atrophy of the reproductive system. Androgens (male sex hormones) administered to female rats during the first 5 days after birth modified the gonadotrophic-releasing mechanisms of the central nervous system so that they became noncyclic, rather than cyclic, in the adult. If androgens were absent from the male during the first 2 days postnatal a cyclic pattern of adult gonadotropin-releasing mechanism was established. The cyclic pattern of gonadotrophin secretion is directly responsible for the oestrous cycle in female rats.

These effects, dependent upon the presence or absence of specific compounds at a critical period of early development, and so permanent in their effects on the long-term organization of behavior and brain function, are properly thought of as chemical imprinting.

The details of the mechanisms by which the presence or absence of androgens during the first few days after birth are translated into a permanent and irrevocable establishment of either a male or a female pattern of gonadotrophin release are in the process of being elaborated; they constitute one of the most exciting chapters in contemporary neuroscience.

Ovulation by the female rat is one event in the 4 to 5 day oestrous cycle. At the beginning of the cycle one of the gonadotrophins, the follicle-stimulating hormone (FSH) secreted by the anterior pituitary, acts on the ovary to stimulate growth of Graffian follicles, which in turn secrete estrogen. The FSH secretion is then shut down, in part as a result of a feedback response to circulating estrogen. Luteinizing hormone (LH), secreted by the pituitary as the next event in the cycle, acts on the Graffian follicle to cause release of the ovum and stimulates the transformation of the disrupted Graffian follicle into the corpus luteum, which secretes progesterone. A feedback by progesterone results in termination of LH secretion. The next cycle begins with a new pulse of FSH secretion.

The cycle is not self-generating, but rather it is dependent upon another event to produce the pulse of FSH. All hormones of the anterior pituitary are under control of the hypothalamus, by means of releasing factors which are transported from the hypothalamus to the pituitary by a branch of the bloodstream known as a portal circulation. The production of releasing factors is accomplished at the axon terminals of specialized neurons in specific nuclei of the hypothalamus, as a result of nerve impulses which originate in the perikarya and travel down the axon (see Chapter 8 for a more complete description of the nerve impulse). This neuronal activity is dependent largely upon the neural organization of the hypothalamic nuclei and partly upon nerve impulses received from other brain regions. Most important, it is cyclic rather than continuous.

The preoptic anterior hypothalamic nuclei (POA) stimulate another hypothalamic area, the ventromedial nuclei, whose neurons produce the individual releasing factors for FSH and LH. The POA region is inherently cyclical at birth with respect to the events outlined above. If at birth androgens or estrogens are present, the POA will mature in such a way that it will become permanently noncyclical by puberty. Androgens are a normal secretion of the male testes starting late in fetal development; estrogens are not secreted by the female ovaries until much later in life. Thus the masculine pattern of POA activity, with respect to control of cyclic gonadotrophin secretion, is imprinted on the normal male brain by androgens. Failure to imprint follows from insufficiency, for any reason, of androgen secretion, and it leads inevitably to a functional female pattern of POA activity in the adult male hypothalamus. Correspondingly, the presence in the neonatal female of either androgens or estrogens during the critical period will imprint a male pattern of acyclic gonadotrophin release on the female hypothalamus.

The search is now vigorously underway for identification of those features of structural and chemical organization which are central to the chemical imprinting process. As is usual at this stage in the elucidation of a problem in science, there are varied observations from several fields which appear to bear on the question at hand. Until the problem is solved it is impossible to say which of these will be productive. Some of the more recent observations are listed below.

1. The effects of abnormal imprinting, as indicated above, include profound changes in sexual behavior. Testosterone propionate (an androgen), when injected into female rats between the 1st and 6th days postnatal, produced sexually unresponsive adults. Injection during the 1st or 2nd day, but not the 6th, also resulted in an abnormally imprinted hypothalamus of the postpubertal female with incapacity to control the oestrous cycle, as indicated above. Thus two systems are imprinted; one, for oestrous which is maximally sensitive during the 1st and 2nd days, and the other for sexual behavior which on more detailed study is found

to be maximally sensitive during the 4th to 6th days after birth.

The relative ineffectiveness of testosterone propionate in impairing the oestrous cycle when given on the 6th day postnatal was found to be true only when the test was made on the postpubertal female, and not with older animals. That is, the effect of imprinting on day 6 was delayed until well after puberty and not lost altogether, indicating that changes in hypothalamic organization continue to occur late in life as a result of the single dose on the 6th day.

2. The impaired oestrous produced by testosterone propionate can be prevented by the simultaneous injection of a wide range of drugs including reserpine, chlorpromazine, progesterone, and phenobarbital. The implication of these observations is that the androgen effect depends upon some ongoing neural activity; if it is changed or suppressed imprinting by androgens cannot occur. In this connection it is interesting to note the possible relevance of some details of "classical" imprinting, as described at the beginning of this chapter. Some of the experimental birds were imprinted to visual or auditory stimuli under the usual conditions; others who were injected with a protein synthesis inhibitor failed to imprint. In a further exploration of the inhibitory effect, it was found that, if the chicks were removed from exposure to light or sound during the few hours the inhibitor was present in effective concentration in the brain and then exposed to imprinting stimuli, normal imprinting occured. Thus the inhibitor disrupted some interaction of the sensory modality (light or sound) with the morphological and neurochemical sites at which imprinting would normally occur. It must be assumed that, when the sensory modality acted on these sites at the same time as did the protein synthesis inhibitor, an abnormal organization of the sites occurred, preventing all future imprinting. The inhibitor alone, in the absence of the sensory modality, merely interferred with protein synthesis, but it did not otherwise damage the organization of the imprinting sites. In the same sense it is possible that the imprint on the hypothalamic site imposed by the androgen required some particular coincident neural or neurochemical events; the drugs tested blocked or altered these events and rendered the androgen, acting alone at the site, ineffective.

3. It can be demonstrated that nerve impulses arising from

other parts of the brain influence the secretion of the releasing factors by the hypothalamus. If all afferent neural connections to the hypothalamus are severed the concentration of releasing factors increases in the hypothalamic nuclei, presumably due to a steady rate of synthesis coupled with diminished release. The other brain areas involved in this control system include the amygdala and hippocampus (both components of the limbic system) as well as the midbrain and cortex. The transmitters involved include at least acetlycholine and dopamine (see Chapter 8).

4. Control of gonadotropin secretion by the pituitary is regulated not only by hypothalamic releasing factors but also by the feedback action of the gonadal hormones on some brain areas. The precise location of such receptive centers for feedback control is not yet known; the search for it is one goal of some research currently in progress. It is known that testosterone is one of the feedback hormones. Recently it has been suggested that testosterone must be metabolically converted to an active hormone and that dihydrotestosterone serves that function. It has been observed that the conversion of testosterone to dihydrotestosterone occurs in two "target" tissues, the prostate and the seminal vesicles, at a much higher rate than in most other tissues. It was postulated that feedback sites in the brain ought to be potent converters of testosterone to its active hormone. The pituitary and hypothalamus have been shown to be more effective than some other brain regions (amygdala and cortex) in accomplishing this conversion.

5. When all afferent nerves to the hypothalamus of the immature male rat are severed, sexual maturation is prevented. When the afferent input to the anterior portion of the hypothalamus is severed, leaving other neural connections intact, sexual maturation occurs more rapidly than in the normal rat. The clear implication of these studies is that the state of hypothalamic activity needed to secrete the gonadotropin-releasing factors is dependent not only upon the intrinsic level of hypothalamic neural activity but also upon both inhibitory and excitatory stimuli from other brain areas.

6. The afferent input to the hypothalamus has been explored in greater detail by destroying very small areas in the rat amyg-

dala. Destruction of the basal portion resulted in an increase in FSH secretion, while an opposite effect was produced by lesions in the medial amygdala. The effectiveness of estradiol to act as a feedback inhibitor of hypothalamic regulation of FSH secretion was diminished as a result of lesions in the basal amygdala, suggesting that the neurochemical site of action of the estrogen is related to the locations in the hypothalamus at which fibers enter from the amygdala.

7. The pineal gland is a very small structure located in the roof of the diencephalon. In the rat it weighs only about 1 milligram. It secretes into the bloodstream several related hormones in varying amounts, depending upon exposure of the animal to light or darkness (Figure 6-1). Serotonin is converted to melatonin

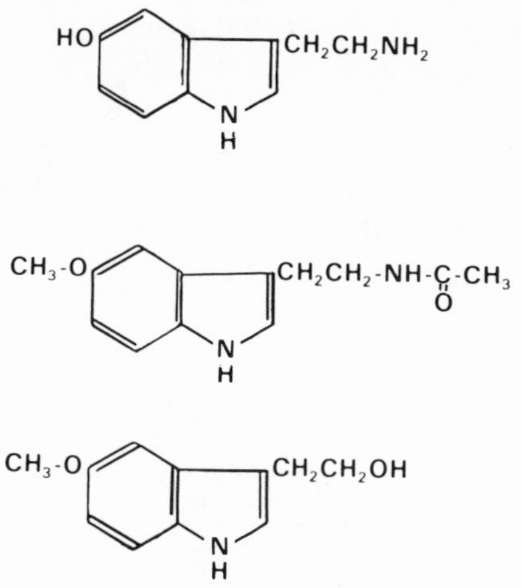

Serotonin

Melatonin

5-methoxytryptophol

Figure 6-1. Some pineal hormones.

during darkness; this diurnal rhythm (Figure 6-2) has been the subject of much intensive study. Melatonin specifically inhibits the secretion of LH, while the related substance 5-methoxytryptophol specifically inhibits FSH secretion. Both substances act on the CNS, rather than directly on the pituitary, to produce their inhibitory effects. The effect of injection of either hormone is to delay puberty in the female rat.

As mentioned above, there is no way of predicting whether these or some totally new observations will provide the clues necessary to elucidate the detailed events of the imprinting phenomenon. The knowledge, once attained, will be most useful as a model for studies of the larger questions of memory storage, neural organization, and the mutual interdependence of neurochemical and environmental events.

The foregoing description of the chemical imprinting of physiological and behavioral patterns can be generalized by focusing attention on the primary physiological events. Hormones present or absent during a short critical period soon after birth will determine, for the life of the animal, whether or not specific cyclical events will occur. In the case of the androgens, as discussed above, the period of the cycle is 4 to 5 days in the rat. The menstrual cycle of 28 days in the human may be subject to similar controls. In the case of the glucocorticosteroids, another group of hormones, an approximately daily cyclic change in blood plasma concentration occurs in both the rat and the human. These circadian cycles are generally found to vary in relation to the

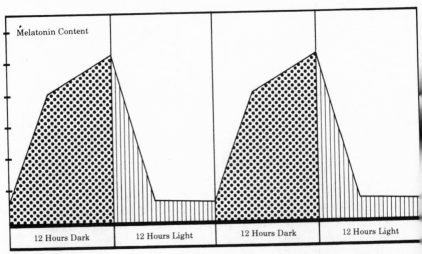

Figure 6-2. Diurnal rhythm in melatonin content of rat pineal.

light-dark cycle of the environment; an example of such a diurnal rhythm has already been illustrated in Figure 6-2.

The glucocorticosteroids are hormones produced by the cortex of the adrenal glands. In man the principal adrenal steroids are 17-hydroxycorticosterone and corticosterone; aldosterone, a hormone with a different physiological function, is one of several other cortical hormones secreted in lesser amounts. The first two listed are designated as glucocorticosteroids because they function to release glucose from the liver and also increase the conversion of amino acids to glucose; the latter effect may be secondary to the inhibition of protein synthesis from amino acids. Aldosterone participates in a system whereby the kidney conserves sodium.

The circadian cycle of changes in the concentration of corticosteroids in the blood plasma of the rat does not become established until the 21st to the 25th days after birth. It has recently been found that this rhythm, characterized by an 8 P.M. concentration that is five times higher than the 8 A.M. concentration, is suppressed in the 30-day-old rat if corticosteroids are administered shortly after birth. Once again there is a brief critical period during which the corticosteroid may be effective; in the species of rat studied the greatest effect was obtained during postnatal days 2 to 4; no effect was obtained during days 12 to 14.

The factors which regulate secretion of corticosteroids are similar to those that regulate estrogens and androgens. A pituitary hormone called adrenocorticotrophic hormone (ACTH) stimulates secretion of a mixture of steroids from the adrenal cortex. The secretion of ACTH is dependent upon a releasing factor liberated from the hypothalamus, which in turn is subject to regulation by other parts of the CNS. There is a circadian rhythm in plasma ACTH; in addition increased secretion by the pituitary commonly results from stress. The stress-induced release of ACTH first develops in the rat much earlier than does the circadian rhythm and thus is thought to be subject to a different set of regulating factors.

At the present time the behavioral correlates of the circadian rhythm in ACTH and corticosteroids remain largely unknown. There are, however, some interesting circadian rhythms in perception that appear to be linked to these substances. In humans, diseases which result in adrenocortical insufficiency are associated with increased perception of the taste of sweet, salt, bitter, and sour stimuli. The accuracy of the perception of these stimuli in such diseases is 100 times greater than that of normal humans. Administration of corticosteroids restores the taste perception to the normal range. In normal humans there is a diurnal variation in the taste threshhold, with the greatest sensitivity occurring in the afternoon and the least in the morning, when the plasma 17-hydroxycorticosteroids are at the highest plasma concentration. Similar observations have been made with respect to recognition of odors, and for auditory acuity as well. The velocity with which impulses travel along nerve axons is increased by 25% in adrenocortical insufficiency. At the same time there is a decreased word discrimination ability, implying that information is lost when there is more rapid signal transmission. Thus the level of responsiveness of several neural systems concerned with transmission and processing of information varies in some way with the plasma concentration of ACTH and corticosteroids; at least with respect to taste, odor, and hearing the variations occur normally in a diurnal rhythm. The possible significance of such variations to other aspects of human behavior remains to be explored, as does the possibility that modification of the circadian rhythm by early exposure to corticosteroids might be expressed in the adult as alterations in expected behavior patterns.

The circadian rhythm in human plasma ACTH and corticosteroid concentration first appears between the ages of 6 months and 4 years. The critical time, if any, for imprinting a noncyclic pattern is not known. It is a true circadian rhythm, tightly linked to the light-dark cycle in the environment. Experimental reversal of the light-dark cycle is followed within 8 days by a compensating change in the plasma hormone levels.

As is the case with imprinting of gonadotrophin-release patterns, the factors that may relate to ACTH and corticosteroid rhythms have been studied in many ways. Removal of the adrenals in experimental animals does not alter the ACTH diurnal cycle; hence the known feedback regulation of ACTH secretion by corticosteroids does not drive the cycle. It has been found that there is a daily rhythm in the hypothalamic content of the corticotropin-releasing factor and that the pattern persists even after removal of the pituitary. The ultimate source of the circadian rhythm is therefore located elsewhere in the CNS. At the present time the hypothalamic and limbic system region is thought to be the site of the cycle, based on the results of experimental lesions in animals. At least three transmitters, acetylcholine, serotonin, and norepinephrine, are required for the neural signals that establish the cycle.

In each of the examples of chemical imprinting discussed above there is a small target region in the hypothalamus which is inherently cyclical at birth with respect to synthesis and secretion of releasing hormones. In the adult the end products of the chain of hormonal stimuli leading from the hypothalamus through the pituitary to some peripheral end organ normally regulate the trophic hormones by negative feedback. In each case, however, their brief presence during a critical period soon after birth disrupts the normal development of the inherently cyclical patterns, with varying behavioral correlates. As neurochemical and neurophysiological research proceeds it becomes increasingly evident that there are many cyclic processes and that the concept of "biological clock" appears to have some reality. Disruption of some of the clocks by chemical imprinting or any other form of early experience could be of profound significance to the adult.

PART TWO

Information Processing

7

The Flow of Information

It is an accepted practice among scientists, when seeking to learn more about an object in nature, to proceed from a qualitative description to quantitative statements. In the case of a biological entity such as a muscle the description begins with what it does and what it is composed of and proceeds to an enumeration of how it utilizes energy and how much work it does. Conceptually at least, it is easy to design experimental approaches to the question of how much work a muscle produces since the concept and experience of physical work is familiar to all of us. Different kinds of questions are required of the brain. One question which has been asked from time to time relates to information. How much information does a brain contain at the end of a lifetime? An answer that is cited frequently is: 10^{20} bits. What this might mean and how the concepts involved might be utilized to construct theoretical models of neural systems are the topics of the first part of this chapter. The second part will deal with the application of these concepts to some specific problems of neural organization and information processing.

The Representation of Information

The general purpose computer, an awesome device that is frequently represented as infallible and virtually omniscient, is constructed of an array of large numbers of an exceedingly simple device, the two-state switch. Such a device, whether it is the clumsy variety that connects or disconnects a light bulb from a supply of electricity or the technological triumph of solid-state microelectronics that controls signal flow in a computer, is the logical equivalent of binary arithmetic.

Quantities can be represented by many number systems, all of which are interconvertible. Each has a symbol for zero and one or more additional symbols. The decimal system with nine nonzero symbols is most familiar to us. The binary system, with a "1" as the only nonzero symbol, is somewhat less familiar. Any integer in the decimal system may have 1 of 10 different values; in the binary system the choice is restricted to "1" or "0." One or zero, true or false, or off or on are logically equivalent statements. Just as decimal numbers can be represented by binary equivalents (for example, the decimal "36" is equivalent to the binary "100100"), it is also true that any statement of logical relations can be represented by a specific array of off-on switches. Furthermore, any information of any kind can be represented by a unique array of off-on switches. The information content of the decimal number "36" in the example above required six binary digits (bits). The particular value assigned to each bit, whether "1" or "0," defined the unique relation between "36" and "100100." The information content of the decimal "36" is therefore six bits. Decimal "43" is represented by another six-bit number, "101011." In the same manner words and other symbols can also be assigned a binary representation, and the total information content of a book, a musical score, or any form of recorded information can be assigned a number of bits.

The estimates of· information recorded in neurons in the brain are based upon the same reasoning. They arose at a time when the all-or-none nature of the nerve impulse and the off-on characteristic of synaptic transmission (see Chapter 8) seemed to be strikingly similar to the binary devices of digital computers. Parenthetically, it should be noted that the brain has always been compared to the most sophisticated technological device of the time: in the eighteenth century the gear-driven clock, wheels-within-wheels-within-wheels, seemed to be an appropriate analogy; at the end of the nineteenth century the telephone switchboard was the obvious model for neural circuitry; and until quite recently the digital computer seemed to many to be a proper model for the brain.

Logical Nets

The assembly of a network of two-state switches into an array that could perform logical functions was aided by the conceptualization of elements of the array, each of which is composed of several such switches. The elements are all variations on the following theme: there is an element proper (the triangle in Figure 7-1A) to which input connections are made (at the left) and from which a single output may be derived. The output may branch, giving rise to multiple inputs to other elements. The inputs may be of two kinds, excitatory and inhibitory. Any parti-

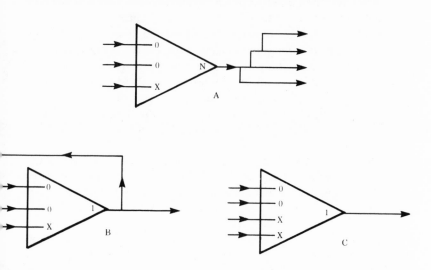

Figure 7-1. Representation of neural net elements. An inhibitory input is represented by the symbol, "X"; an excitatory input by the symbol "O."

cular element is described by a threshold number, N, such that, when the number of excitatory inputs exceeds the number of inhibitory inputs by N, the element "fires." Firing or nonfiring at any specific time is equivalent to the "1" or "0" of a binary digit, to the closing or opening of a two-state switch, or to any other on-off device that one cares to imagine.

Each element is assumed to take the same time to fire and to be refractory over a time interval which is the same for all elements. There is one variation, described as a loop element, having the additional property that an output branch may return as an input. The simplest result of this return path occurs when the loop element contains one excitatory and one inhibitory input and a threshold of $N=1$. Then an excitatory input results in repetitive refiring of the element, via the return loop from the output, until the process is stopped by an inhibitory input. This is the simplest representation of a reverberating circuit. Obviously any number of elements can be assembled in a chain, with the last one refiring the first, given appropriate values of N for each element. Such a circuit constitutes a memory (see Figure 7-1B).

One particular element is sufficiently general so that by appropriate combinations with others of the same kind it is possible to derive the various connectives, such as "inclusive or," "and," or "not" of Boolean algebra. It consists of an element of threshold $N=1$ to which are attached two permanently activated excitatory inputs and two inhibitory inputs (see Figure 7-1C). This element fires unless both inhibitory inputs are activated at the same time.

A net of elements of the types described above contains input elements, interior elements, and output elements. Because all of the elements are synchronized (have discrete times at which any or all are permitted to fire), the history of a net can be represented by a time-element matrix, where the columns of the matrix are individual input elements, and the successive rows are instants of time reading back from the present. At each location a "1" or a "0" is entered, signifying the firing or nonfiring of a particular input element at a particular instant in time.

Artificial Intelligence

Given the availability of such nets, it was of more than passing interest to explore their capabilities for information processing at a relatively high level of sophistication. The first constructions were designed to explore the problem of pattern recognition. We easily distinguish symbols such as "*H*" from "*N*." One way to approach the problem of learning how a brain is organized to make such distinctions is to build several varieties of artificial intelligence automata and examine the relation of performance to built-in operating principles. The general approach has been to transduce the pattern by means of appropriate sensors into a set of input signals. These signal sets were then compared with sets of signals derived from patterns which had previously been introduced as knowns into the memory of the device.

The response was required as a statement as to whether the new input signal set could be identified as similar to any set previously stored in memory. The programs for evaluating the degree of correspondence generally functioned by listing the probability that particular properties would occur in a given known pattern. The weight, or importance, of a particular property in the overall evaluation process can be assigned a constant value throughout, or it can vary as the device evaluates successive unknowns and information concerning the correctness of the evaluation is fed back. When the weight is made to vary in this manner, the program learns the desired response. To give a very simple example of weight in pattern recognition, consider that the upper case letters, *A,E,F,H,I,K,L,* and *M* had been converted to signal sets and introduced into memory as knowns. Each might be represented as a construction of three or four straight lines with vertical, horizontal, or diagonal elements. Initially each of the descriptors just listed might have been assigned equal weight. Now introduce as an unknown the letter *N* and ask the device for an identification. There are three straight lines, composed of verticals and a diagonal, but no horizontal. The response might have been that the new pattern is most like the letter *K*, which also has three lines composed of verticals and diagonals but no horizontal. The error was based on giving too much weight to the three lines, which are common among all the knowns. As a result of the first error, the program would randomly try to adjust the weight of each descriptor. When the three-line descriptor is reduced in weight, fewer errors will result. This simple example does not do justice to the complexity of such learning devices, but it does illustrate the close correspondence between the use of computers for studies of artificial intelligence and the underlying concept of neural structure. Each requires a sensory input, a means of processing and categorizing information, a memory, and a feedback from the environment so that learning can occur. For a considerable period of time the apparent digital nature of the nerve impulse provided an alluring comparison to the efficiency of binary logic and digital computers. More recent information about the variety of synaptic junctions (Chapter 1) and the wide range of transmitters (Chapter 8) has led to the understanding that the brain must be described in terms of systems far more complex than those based on binary logic. Nevertheless, the concepts of neural nets as first elaborated for artificial intelligence automata have proved useful in understanding the information-processing capabilities of limited regions of the nervous system.

Neural Models

The elements of Figure 7-1 have sometimes been referred to as "formal neurons." The entrance points at the left of each element are taken as equivalent to synaptic junctions; the body of the element represents a perikaryon; and the output line is the efferent axon. The use of such elements as components in artificial intelligence automata has usually required the assumption that each element has an unchanging and error-free response. Thus each successive input to a given "synapse" will always change the threshold by exactly one unit, the threshold requirement itself will not change, and the output pulse, obtained when each element fires, will always have the same magnitude and duration.

A system composed of elements of this kind is said to be deterministic. In the case where at least one feature is not known precisely at any given instant, for example if the threshold of an element is five 80% of the time and six 20% of the time, the system is described as probabilistic. The debate between probability and determinism, which is an ancient one in science and philosophy, has apparently attracted new interest as a result of its application to this challenging field. In its simplest form it is usually stated as follows: if the same real neuron is repeatedly exposed to the same stimulus, will it always produce the same response? The difficulty here is that the question is unreal. At least with respect to its neurochemical structure, the data summarized so far in this book should make it clear that the neuron cannot be said to be the same at any two instants in time. So also with respect to the storage of information, which must occur in many CNS neurons (see Chapter 9), it is likely that the neuron must change throughout its life history. Nevertheless many attempts have been made to model the performance of some aspects of the CNS on the basis that the neurons involved are deterministic, while other equally vigorous attempts have been made to design reliable models composed of unreliable components. "Reliable" is always taken to mean that the whole system produces almost the same response when presented with the same stimulus. An example of each viewpoint will be presented.

The earliest attempt to achieve reliability with a net of imperfect cells made extensive use of the principle of redundancy. A given input signal would be presented in parallel paths to many receiving cells. Even though some cells might respond with gross errors in signal handling, it was assumed that most would perform as required. The output signal was obtained as the majority vote of all of the cells. Since there is apparently an extensive redundancy in the CNS (see Chapter 9), this concept appeared to relate the model to the real organism. In a newer and more sophisticated approach it is assumed that each cell in the net receives information from a small subgroup and that each cell in the subgroup computes a different function of the information it receives. Parts of the many computation programs are stored at various locations within the net, and the individual computations are encoded at one location and transmitted elsewhere, where they are decoded. The individual component cells must be complex in order to be able to store both codes and programs. Maintaining stability of such a system requires extensive feedback, locally for the modification of synapses as well as externally for overall correction. The feedback results in adaptability, which is a general feature of a class of neural nets known as perceptrons.

Some of these concepts are implicit in the following analysis

of the function of the cerebellar cortex. The microscopic structure of this part of the CNS is not unlike that of the cerebral
cortex (Chapter 1) in that there are several distinct cellular layers.
The layer closest to the surface, the molecular layer, is composed
largely of dendritic branches and unmyelinated axonal branches.
Just below there is a single row of Purkinje cells whose extensive
dendritic branches penetrate the molecular layer. The myelinated
axons of the Purkinje cells are directed inward from the surface,
projecting either to nuclei deep within the cerebellum, as association fibers to other Purkinje cells, or occasionally directly through
the cerebellum to other parts of the CNS. In any case they constitute the only pathway by which information leaves the cerebellar
cortex. Just below the Purkinje cells there is a dense cellular
region called the granular layer, from which axons of the granular
cells run upward into the molecular layer and continue as
branches parallel to the surface.

Afferent fibers are of two kinds. There are climbing fibers,
which branch extensively and appear to be in close contact with
the dendritic tree of the Purkinje cells. Some of them may originate from a nucleus in the medulla called the inferior olive (see
Figure 1-4). The second category is known as mossy fibers. They
give off some branches which make contact with the dendrites of
the granule cells and others which apparently synapse with
Purkinje cells. They may originate from the spinal cord, the
inferior olive, or the pontine nuclei.

The model of cerebellar function assumes that each cell in
the inferior olive sends climbing fibers to only one Purkinje cell.
During learning it is postulated that each olivary cell responds to
an instruction, originating from the cerebral cortex, for a muscle
movement and that the flow of information occurs from the
cerebral cortex to the olive to the cerebellar Purkinje cell and then
to the effector cell for muscle action. At the same time the
Purkinje cell is supplied with information about the context in
which the olivary cell fired, by means of the mossy fiber input.
The contextual information is learned as a result of an unspec-
ified alteration in a synaptic region of the Purkinje cell. After
learning, another signal, which contains only context and is transmitted through the mossy fiber, can fire the Purkinje cell. Each
Purkinje cell is postulated to be able to learn a large number of

contexts; hence the output of such a cell is not readily predicted in a deterministic fashion.

In contrast to this model of variable cell function a model proposed for the olfactory system is strongly oriented toward the deterministic outlook. The olfactory system of the cat begins in the nasal mucosa with about 100 million receptor neurons whose axons constitute the primary olfactory nerve. Terminal branches of the axons cover the surface of the olfactory bulb, which is located on the basal surface of the cerebral hemisphere. The surface of the bulb contains masses of synaptic endings, glomeruli, which are surrounded by periglomerular cells. Below this there is a layer of mitral and tufted cells and below that another layer of granule cells. The output from the olfactory bulb consists of the bundles of axons arising from the mitral cells. This fiber bundle, the lateral olfactory tract, terminates in the prepyriform cortex, which is composed of a surface layer of pyramidal cells, below which there is an intermediate layer of granule cells and then a deep layer of pyramidal cells. Most of the axons of the deep cellular layer, which constitute the output of this region, are distributed widely in the basal and lateral forebrain and in the hypothalamus; some axons feed back to the olfactory bulb.

The essential hypothesis of this model is that there are populations of neurons, where each unit in the population is extensively interconnected with the others, where there is a common input, and where the output of each unit is either inhibitory or excitatory. That is, a whole population functions predictably to produce one kind of output, regardless of input. The interconnections within a population result in positive feedback; a small incoming signal is rapidly amplified by the neurons within an excitatory population, while a signal entering an inhibitory population is rapidly attenuated.

The model postulates that the periglomerular neurons are an excitatory population, as are the mitral and tufted cell populations. The granule cells are said to be an inhibitory population. Granule cells in the prepyriform cortex are also inhibitory, whereas the two pyramidal layers are excitatory. The deep pyramidal layer feeds back to the granule cells in the olfactory bulb and also provides output to other parts of the CNS. The model is consistent with the postulate that varying input from the olfactory mucosa can be converted to a controlled oscillatory output, representing information about the odors which come into contact with the receptor cells.

Neural Organization

The Eye of the Horseshoe Crab

There is a relatively simple neural network in the eye of Limulus, the horseshoe crab, that has been the subject of extensive experimental investigations. The image of any object that the eye sees is focused on a single layer of photoreceptors by the lens. Limulus has a compound eye, with many lenses. Each lens sees a small portion of the object and focuses on a few photoreceptors. However, the visual fields of adjacent receptors overlap, as illustrated in Figure 7-2. The row of nine receptors in the diagram see

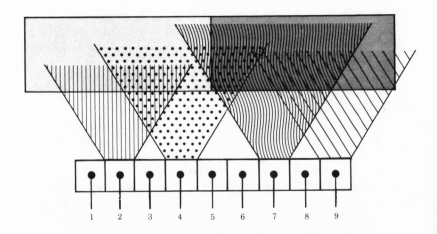

Figure 7-2. The overlap of the visual fields of photoreceptors.

different parts of a bar which is a light color at the left and dark at the right. The visual fields of each receptor are contained within the lines drawn from the surface of the receptor to the object. Receptor number 4 is shown as receiving information from the light and dark regions of the bar. The perikaryon of each receptor generates a potential whose magnitude depends upon the amount of light falling on it. The potential is coded into a burst of impulses which traverses the axon with a frequency that is related to the size of the generator potential. The bundle of axons carries this information to the CNS. If there were no modifications of this circuit, the sharp contrast between the light and dark regions of the object would be lost because of the mixed information obtained by receptors focused on the boundary region. The magnitude of the potentials occurring in receptors located directly below their visual fields on the object is illustrated in Figure 7-3.

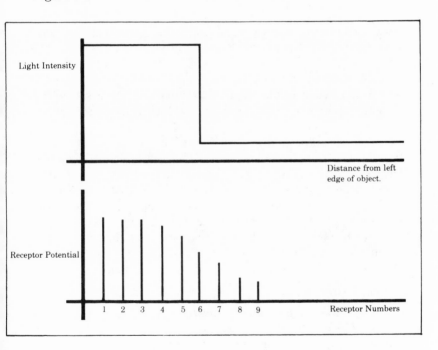

Figure 7-3. The uncorrected generator potentials in individual receptors.

This loss of precision is overcome by a process known as lateral inhibition. The axon of each receptor gives off branches to its nearest neighbors, as illustrated in Figure 7-4 for receptor. The lateral axonal branches inhibit the perikarya of the receptors with

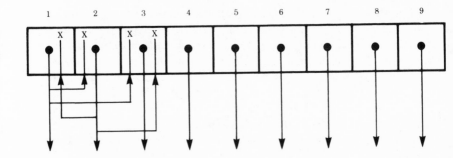

Figure 7-4. Schematic drawing of lateral inhibition. Branches of the axons of each photoreceptor feed back to adjacent and nearby receptors. The feedback inputs are inhibitory, designated by the symbol "X."

which they synapse. The inhibition depends upon the size of the generator potential in the perikaryon which is the source of the lateral fiber.

Thus receptor number 6 of Figure 7-3 would retain the illustrated potential only until the feedback signals obtained from the large potential in receptor number 4 and 5 are subtracted from its initial value. The resultant distribution of potentials is illustrated in Figure 7-5. This simple computation, which makes use of the differing polarities of excitatory and inhibitory potentials (see Chapter 8), actually results in a sharpening of the information about the border region. Although the circuitry is illustrated for Limulus, similar considerations apply to the human eye.

Striatal Neurocircuits

The preceding example dealt with computation in a localized group of neurons; the following example will illustrate circuitry in large systems of neural structures.

The corpus striatum is an essential part of the extrapyramidal system (see Chapter 1). Part of its output is directed toward the red nucleus and the nuclei of the reticular formation. The control of large muscle movements originates from the striatal output. The organization of such controlled activity has been postulated to have the following characteristics: a feedback function which regulates postural position; a "set" function which

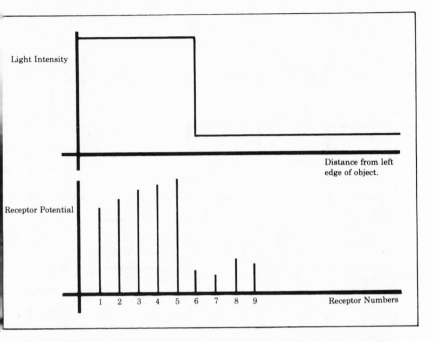

Figure 7-5. Corrected generator potentials in individual receptors. The corrections occur as the result of lateral inhibition.

prepares the CNS and the muscles involved for impending movement; and a "trigger" function which initiates the movement.

The block diagram of Figure 7-6 outlines the interrelations of the major neural systems involved in the feedback control. The immediate output for muscle movement originates from the paleostriatum (the globus pallidus). At the muscle end of the system, proprioceptive input, describing the instantaneous position and movement of the muscle, is fed back via the brainstem and the thalamus to the neostriatum (the caudate and putamen). Stimulation of this region causes an inhibitory output signal to be sent to the globus pallidus, whose muscle-stimulating activity is thereby diminished. Opposed to this regulation, however, there is another feedback loop from the globus pallidus to the substantia nigra to the neostriatum and back to the globus pallidus. As indicated in Figure 7-6, the excitatory signal from the globus

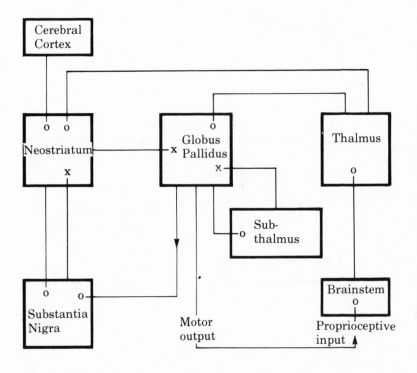

Figure 7-6. A model of some striatal and related circuits. Inhibitory inputs are symbolized by "X" and excitatory inputs by "O."

pallidus stimulates the substantia nigra to send an inhibitory signal
to the neostriatum. Thus the inhibition of the globus pallidus
is in turn inhibited, with the result that the output of the globus
pallidus tends to increase. However, still another feedback circuit
between the subthalamus and the globus pallidus limits this increase. Signals from the thalamus and cerebral cortex also stimulate the neostriatum, thus inhibiting the globus pallidus.

   These interrelations, even at this level of description, are
obviously too complicated to allow a conclusion as to what the
resultant activity would be. One of the principal difficulties is that
a model of this sort is essentially similar to the one outlined above
for the olfactory system, in that the use of blocks to represent

neuronal regions implies populations of neurons having unitary activity. There is no way of knowing, for example, whether any individual neuron in the globus pallidus, which sends an axonal branch to a particular neuron in the substantia nigra, in turn receives a synaptic input from the same neuron in the neostriatum which is in synaptic contact with the neuron from the substantia nigra. Thus such models, although useful to the extent that they lead to further experimentation, have limited value in describing the flow of information from neuron to neuron.

All the models discussed in this chapter have implied a signal code between neurons that is based on the frequency of impulses traveling along an axon. None of the models specifically makes use of the chemical coding that is implicit in the multiplicity of neurotransmitters available to the CNS. The problem can be stated as follows: if two closely adjacent regions of a perikaryon receive impulses at the rate of 20 per second through separate synapses, is the information content at each synaptic junction the same or does the perikaryon have any way of differentiating between the two signals? The following chapter will deal with this aspect of information flow in the CNS.

8

Chemical Communication Between Neurons

OF THE SEVERAL modes of organization available to the more than 10 billion neurons in the human brain, the one dependent upon specific chemical events has recently been subject to the most intense investigation, for it is in this area that an increase in knowledge of the basic molecular chemistry of the nerve impulse has seemed to correlate well with the rationale for the therapeutic use of drugs to modify behavior.

As an information-processing device, the brain is capable of storage, retrieval, transmission, and data processing. Transmission—the movement of information from one neuron to another—is recognized to occur in at least three distinct steps. The first, the action potential, is electrochemical in nature. The second, synaptic transmission, requires the movement of a relatively few transmitter molecules across the synaptic cleft. The third, postsynaptic depolarization or hyperpolarization, begins with a structural reorganization at receptor sites and terminates in an electrochemical change.

Electrochemistry—the association of electrochemical events

with chemical changes—is a rather complex field of study. However, insofar as the action potential is concerned, the required concepts are rather simple and are contained in the following hypothetical experiment.

Divide a container of water into right and left halves by inserting a thin plastic partition. Place a small quantity of NaCl in the left half and 10 times that amount in the right half. Put wires in each half and connect a voltmeter between the wires. Now quickly, but without agitating the solution, remove the plastic barrier. The voltmeter will indicate an initial reading of a few millivolts, with the left half being negative. After some time the electrical potential between the two sides will disappear because of the slow diffusion of ions out of the more concentrated region. It is a fundamental occurance in nature that all differences tend to disappear whenever interactions are allowed to occur spontaneously, that is, without the intervention of energy from an external source.

The initial voltmeter reading observed in the preceding hypothetical experiment was due to the dissociation of NaCl into the positive and negative ions, Na^+ and Cl^-, and the more rapid movement of some of the Cl ions, after removal of the barrier, to the left side.

A modification of the hypothetical experiment is instructive. Suppose that in place of the initial impermeable barrier there was a different barrier containing a number of very small holes, and further suppose that these holes somehow resisted the flow of the Cl^- ions but allowed a sizable flow of Na^+ ions. In such a case the electrical potential across this semipermeable barrier would be about 58 millivolts, with the left side positive. Again the potential would be due to the movement of a small number of ions between the initially neutral compartments. The net movement would result in the "downhill" transfer of a few Na^+ ions from the more concentrated right half to the less concentrated left half, thereby producing an excess of positive charge in the left side.

The movement of Na^+ ions from one region to another is referred to as a sodium current, and it constitutes an electrical current just as surely as does the movement of electrons through the metal wires in any electrical appliance.

The imaginary semipermeable barrier has some real-life

equivalents. The interior contents of every cell in living organisms are separated from the surroundings by a specialized region known as a membrane. Almost without exception, all cell membranes are semipermeable, in the sense that they allow some substances to penetrate easily and others only with difficulty, if at all. Membranes from differing kinds of cells vary with respect to the substances that may penetrate. All, however, will allow Na^+ and K^+, the ion of the closely related element potassium to penetrate at any time. All, that is, except for the membranes of neurons.

Neuronal membranes have the specialized ability to choose the time at which they will allow either a rapid or a slow flow of Na^+ and K^+ ions. How they do this, and what the consequences are, is one-third of the story of how nerve cells communicate with each other.

The Action Potential

An action potential is a reversal of the normal resting potential that occurs across an axonal membrane. It can be initiated experimentally by electrical or chemical stimulation or physiologically by certain changes in the membranes that surround the body and dendrites of the neuron. In the latter case it is first detected at the region known as the axon hillock, where the axon emerges from the cell body. Once initiated it is self-propagating, traveling down the axon in wavelike fashion through its many branches to the synaptic regions that constitute the end of each branch.

The resting potential across the semipermeable membranes of perikarya and axons arises from a concentration difference between Na^+ and K^+ ions, as was true for the hypothetical experiment described above. However, a fuller understanding of the physiological resting potential requires a more detailed description of the cell body and its surrounding fluid.

The interior contents of all living cells contain a variety of substances ranging in particle size from the relatively small ions such as H_3O^+, K^+, Cl^-, HCO_3^- to macromolecules whose particle size and weight may be hundreds of thousands, or sometimes even millions, of times greater than those of the simple ions. Because these macromolecules are so much larger than the diameter of the pores in cell membranes they are almost entirely retained within the cell. Frequently a macromolecule will bear an electrical charge, and most often this charge will be negative. The requirement that the bulk contents of the cell be electrically neutral can be met by accumulating positive ions in sufficient number to neutralize the total anionic charge of the macromolecule. It is important to recognize that this is a statistical requirement; no single cation needs to be bound forever to the macromolecule, although such binding is not precluded. Thus on the average a certain fraction of the soluble cations are restricted to the interior of the cell, with the result that the total cation concentration inside the cell is greater than in the surrounding medium. This requirement alone gives rise to a difference in charge between the inside and outside of the cell, known as a Donnan potential. However, there is nothing in the nature of the Donnan potential, as outlined above, that would result in a selective intracellular accumulation of one cation with respect to another. Nevertheless this is in fact what usually occurs. The intracellular K^+ of most cells is about 20 times more concentrated than the extracellular K^+, and, correspondingly, the intracellular Na^+ concentration may be only 1/20 of the extracellular Na .

As has already been observed in connection with the hypothetical experiment, such differences in concentration tend to disappear unless an external energy source intervenes to maintain them. The mechanism by which such huge differences in concentration are maintained has been extensively investigated by scientists for many years. The nature of the problem has been formalized by assigning to it the terms "active transport" or "uphill transport," which imply that an energy source must be coupled to the movement of ions across the cell membrane in order to produce such an unlikely distribution.

Although the metabolic energy of all animals ultimately derives from the oxidation of foods, the way in which the energy is applied varies with the nature of the requirement. In the case of active transport there is good reason to believe that ATP, a high-energy compound composed of phosphate groups combined with a nucleotide, and ATP-ase, the enzyme which releases phosphate from it, are part of a membrane transport system known as the sodium pump. It is supposed that this system has a particular spatial organization within the membrane which favors the outward movement of Na$^+$and the coupled inward movement of K$^+$.

The result of the normal operation of the sodium pump, then, is to produce an intracellular K$^+$ concentration some 20 times higher than the extracellular K$^+$, with an inverse relation for Na$^+$. The resting neuronal membrane is only slightly permeable to Na$^+$, but much more permeable to K$^+$. Thus movement of a small number of K$^+$ ions out of the cell, in the direction of the "downhill" concentration gradient, leaves the interior contents negatively charged by about 50 to 100 millivolts. This potential difference occurs across a membrane which is 50 to 100 hundred-millionths of a centimeter thick. The potential gradient across the resting membrane is thus of the order of 100,000 volts per centimeter—a very intense field.

The resting membrane therefore owes its potential to the prior action of the sodium pump, which had already pumped Na$^+$ and K$^+$ ions uphill against concentration gradients. Much more rapid events characterize the action potential. At the time an action potential is initiated the neuronal membrane becomes suddenly permeable to Na$^+$. Since the Na$^+$ is concentrated extracellularly, the immediate result of the permeability change, which may be likened to an opening of the gates, is to allow a downhill movement of Na$^+$ to the intracellular region of lower Na$^+$ concentration. This sodium current, which is a movement of positive charge into the cell, reverses the resting potential within about 1/2 millisecond. It must be emphasized at this time that only a few of the external Na$^+$ ions have crossed the membrane and that the intra-extracellular concentration difference is essentially unchanged. For reasons which have not yet been determined, the membrane now reverts to its state of sodium impermeability and the sodium current is shut off. At about this time the permeability of the membrane to K$^+$ increases greatly, and an outward downhill movement of K$^+$ occurs, requiring about 1 to 1.5 milliseconds. Thus positive charge is carried out of the cell and the membrane regains its resting potential. The region of the membrane directly adjacent to the site of the changes just described, probably stimulated by the neighboring flow of current, then undergoes the same cycle of permeability changes and current flow. In this manner a wave of positive charge **moves** along the axon and through each of its many branches toward its terminal.

The rate at which the wave front moves is related to the diameter of the axon. It is as slow as 1/10 meter per second in narrow unmyelinated axons and may be greater than 100 meters per second in large myelinated axons. The effect of myelin is related to its apparent insulating properties. Myelinated axons contain relatively long segments of myelin interspersed with short unmyelinated segments. An action potential occuring at the unmyelinated node is not regenerated throughout the myelinated region, but in effect it jumps rapidly to the next node, where regeneration occurs.

The action potential is customarily represented as an "all-or-none" phenomenom. Either the depolarizing stimulus is insufficient to initiate an action potential, or it is great enough, if applied at the same site on the axon, to produce an action potential whose size and shape cannot be altered by further increasing the strength of the stimulus. The "all-or-none" law would thus seem to imply that the information content of any one action potential occurring along one particular axon is not substantially different from one occurring along another axon.

Such a conclusion, however, would not be in accord with the following considerations. The maximum amplitude of an action potential is dependent upon the sodium current, which in turn is preset by the energy supply systems which have established the resting ratio of intra-extracellular Na^+. Thus the background metabolic state of a particular neuron will be one of the determinants of the amplitude of its axon's action potential. Not only variations in size, shape, and proximity to nutrient supply but also variation in the instantaneous state of activity produced by the ebb and flow of incoming nerve impulses can be expected to alter the moment-to-moment metabolic state of any neuron. Thus from this point of view alone the amplitude of the action potential will be expected to depend upon the structure and metabolic state of the source neuron.

The duration of the action potential will depend upon how rapidly the potassium current restores the axonal membrane to its resting state. This in turn can be expected to vary as the potassium transport system in the membrane varies in response to slow changes in the chemical structure of the membrane as well as in response to externally applied agents such as rapidly acting drugs. The speed of propagation of the action potential is dependent upon the diameter of the axon and upon the presence or absence of myelin. At least in the case of the demyelinating diseases it will be obvious that, as long as the axon itself remains intact, a dramatic decrease in progagation speed will have occurred. More subtle changes in the chemical structure of the myelin, especially near the terminal branches where myelinated axonal segments may be contiguous with unmyelinated segments, could also affect the propagation speed.

To summarize briefly, then, the action potential may vary in size and shape from moment to moment and over a longer time period in propagation speed as well. If such variations were random, in effect "noise," then the information-processing system of the brain would contain a way to reduce their effects. If, on the other hand, they were not random they might very well constitute useful information. The import of such variations remains to be explored.

Synaptic Transmission

The action potential may be thought of as a wave of positive charge traveling within the axon to its terminal branches. At the terminal this self-propagating wave comes to a halt and the transmission of the nerve impulse takes another form. Briefly what happens is this: the positive wave causes the release of a small number of organic molecules which in turn carry the message of the action potential across the synaptic cleft and onto the dendrites and body of the next neuron.

The detailed knowledge of which molecules serve as transmitters, how they are synthesized, stored, and metabolized, and how their actions can be impaired or augmented by therapeutic drugs has been acquired as a result of intensive investigation by many scientists in the recent past.

Acetylcholine was the first substance to be recognized as a transmitter in the central nervous system. It is synthesized by adding an assembly of atoms known as an acetyl group to choline, a strongly charged organic cation. The acetyl group is transferred from a coenzyme called acetyl Co-A, under the influence of choline acetyltransferase, an enzyme found in active form in the cytoplasm of certain nerve fibers known as cholinergic fibers. Once synthesized, acetylcholine is stored in packets in the nerve terminals. Specific numbers of packets are then released from a terminal upon arrival of the positive wave of the action potential. This phenomenom is known as quantal release.

The effect of acetylcholine and other transmitters on the postsynaptic membrane will be discussed in more detail below. At this point it is important to note that, when the transmitter quanta have reached their target site, approximately 300 hundred-millionths of a centimeter distant from the site of release, they produce an alteration in membrane permeability. It is essential that such a change be transitory so that the effect of later nerve impulses may also be recognized. There are at least two mechanisms by which this requirement can be met. The first is diffusion away from the target site, presumably followed by a reversal of the permeability effects of the transmitter. The second is enzymatic conversion. For acetylcholine the second mechanism is by far the more important. The enzyme involved, acetylcholinesterase, splits acetylcholine into its two constituents, choline and acetate. Acetylcholinesterase is a rapidly acting enzyme. It has been estimated that it can hydrolyze acetylcholine fast enough to allow a target site to respond to individual waves of a transmitter arriving at the rate of 1,000 per second.

Consistent with this high rate of enzyme activity, it has been observed that acetylcholine is usually found at the terminals of myelinated fibers. Since the nerve impulse is conducted most rapidly along such axons it seems clear that cholinergic transmission—the utilization of acetylcholine as the transmitter at the synaptic cleft—is specialized for those informational processes requiring the most rapid rate of transmission.

A substantially different mechanism for recovery from the effects of a transmitter exists for a group of substances known as "biogenic amines." In this case the predominant mechanism for removal of the active transmitter is by re-uptake, which is a return diffusion from the postsynaptic membrane to the presynaptic membrane, followed by a reincorporation into the nerve terminal. Since such a return involves movement into the terminal against a concentration gradient, energy is required, and an "amine pump" is presumed to operate. The re-uptake mechanism is slower than the enzymatic mechanism, and thus it must serve a different category of informational requirement, perhaps characterized less by rapid barrages of short impulses than by other attributes of the action potential.

The major amine transmitters in the brain are noradrenalin, dopamine, and serotonin. The first two are members of a class of compounds called catecholamines; the third is a member of the indolealkylamine group (See Figure 8-1). For several years these substances have been implicated in the regulation of normal and abnormal mood states, and alterations in their metabolism and distribution in the brain, as inferred by studying metabolites appearing in body fluids, have indeed seemed to correlate with manic-depressive illness. A more detailed account will be presented in Chapter 13; for the present it is useful to survey the extensive neurochemical knowledge related to these substances.

Each of the amines is synthesized within a neuron. Within any one neuron only one synthetic path is active. Precursors of each transmitter, accumulated in a perikaryon, are transported along each of the many axonal branches to each terminal of that neuron, where a sequence of enzyme-catalyzed reactions leads to

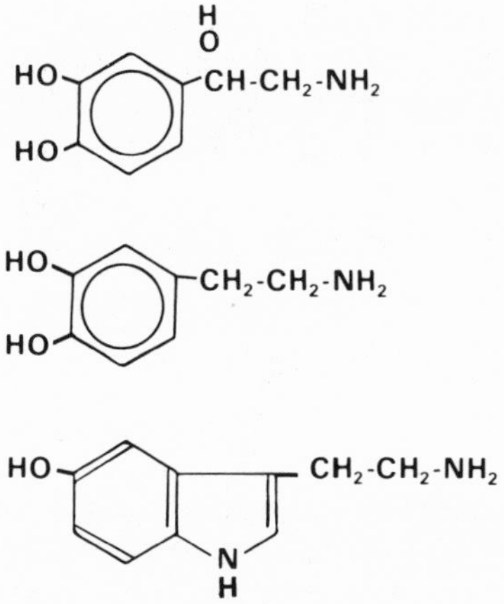

Norephinephrine (noradrenalin)

Dopamine

Serotonin

Figure 8-1. Some amine transmitters.

the final product. Overproduction is regulated along the synthetic route and also by metabolic enzymes which convert any excess into inert substances. Finally the products are stored at discrete locations in the terminal. Some storage sites serve as reserve pools while others are responsive to an arriving action potential.

Dopamine, more accurately known as dihydroxyphenyl-ethylamine, is produced from 1-tyrosine, an amino acid. The first step requires the enzyme tyrosine hydroxylase, which adds a hydroxyl group to the aromatic ring of tyrosine. The second step, with the aid of the enzyme dopa decarboxylase, effects a removal of the carboxyl group from 1-dopa, the intermediate amino acid. The product is dopamine (Figure 8-2). In another population of

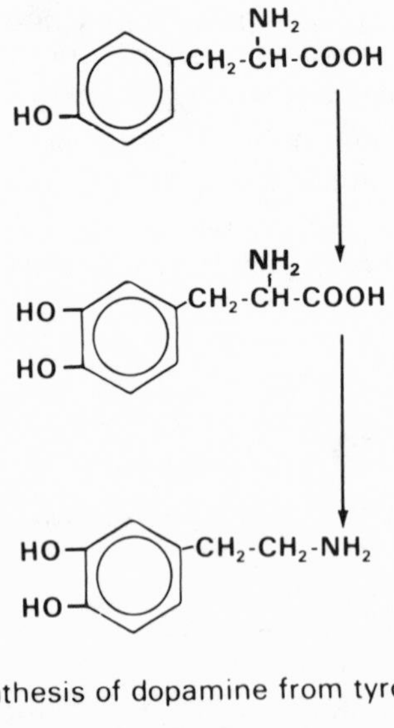

Figure 8-2. Synthesis of dopamine from tyrosine.

neurons an additional enzyme, dopamine beta hydroxylase, converts dopamine to noradrenalin. Noradrenalin, by the process of feedback inhibition, can limit the activity of tyrosine hydroxylase, which is the slowest enzyme in the system producing noradrenalin.

All of these enzymes occur in nerve terminals and are thus

well situated to regulate the concentration of the transmitters within the terminals. A final regulatory process is imposed by monoamine oxidase, an enzyme which converts any of the amine transmitters to inert products by removing the amino group.

Serotonin, the third amine transmitter, is produced by a similar sequence of reactions from the amino acid l-tryptophan. The first step, under the influence of the enzyme tryptophan hydroxylase, leads to the intermediate amino acid, 5-hydroxy tryptophan. This in turn, with the aid of the enzyme amino acid decarboxylase, loses a carboxyl group. The product is serotonin. Its level in the nerve terminal can also be regulated by monoamine oxidase.

Although the relatively rapid regulation of transmitter concentrations within the nerve terminals is accomplished with the enzymes described above and with drugs that interact with these enzymes (see Chapter 11), there are important background regulatory factors. First, brain tyrosine levels are dependent upon total body concentrations which in turn are regulated in part by an enzyme found in the liver, tyrosine transaminase. Brain tryptophan levels are similarly dependent upon the concentration in the blood, which is responsive to the activity of pyrrolase, an enzyme in the liver which converts most of the tryptophan to formylkynurinine, from which a variety of other metabolites, including nicotinic acid, are formed. Pyrrolase activity is elevated by an increase in the blood levels of the adrenocorticosteroids, with the result that brain tryptophan and serotonin decrease when these steroids are injected into experimental animals.

Secondly, movement of the amino acid precursors and enzymes from the perikaryon to its axonal terminal depends upon the process of axoplasmic flow—the movement of cytoplasm along the axon. It has recently been found that there are several rates of flow, some very slow and others relatively rapid. Although it is not yet known what factors regulate the axoplasmic flow rates, we can suppose that transmitter concentrations in terminals might be responsive to alterations in the flow rates.

There are therefore a number of factors which regulate the levels of the three amine transmitters within at least three populations of neurons. The information content of an action potential is ultimately expressed by transmitter release. If more or less than the normal quantal release occurs as a result of altered transmitter levels, the state of activity of the brain has been altered.

In addition to the substances described above there is substantial evidence for a transmitter role for several amino acids, particularly glutamic acid, aspartic acid, gamma aminobutyric acid, and glycine. Additionally another amine, histamine, which can be produced in the brain from the amino acid histidine, is also suspected to have a transmitter function. There is no reason to believe that this completes the list; evidence for the transmitter function of other substances is likely to accumulate as research proceeds.

To summarize thus far: at least four, and perhaps nine, substances can be presumed to function as transmitters of information between the terminal of one nerve and the cell body of another. Each is associated with specific populations of neurons serving specialized functions in the overall organization of the brain. It is not unlikely that a single neuron may be stimulated by terminals belonging, for example, to other neurons whose transmitters are acetylcholine, noradrenaline, and gamma aminobutyric acid. Each transmitter will exert a different effect from the others, thereby providing a means by which the receiving neuron can recognize the kind of neuron with which it is in communication at any instant. The details of the response mechanism available to the receiving neuron are the final third of the story of how nerve cells communicate with each other.

Postsynaptic Response

When transmitter molecules move across the synaptic cleft and come into contact with the postsynaptic membrane they initiate changes in that membrane which ultimately increase or reduce the resting potential. The first event is widely assumed to be a combination with a receptor molecule. Although no researcher doubts that it will come, the unassailable proof of such combinations and the identification of specific receptors has yet to be accomplished. The reason, in part at least, is related to the underlying hypothesis. The receptor-transmitter combination is required to lead to a transient, reversible change in the physicochemical structure of the membrane. The requirement for reversibility means that either the receptor-transmitter combination must break away from the membrane and be subject to further action to insure against recombination or else the combination itself must come apart, with subsequent removal or further modification of the transmitter. It has already been pointed out that acetylcholine is subject to cleavage by the enzyme acetylcholinesterase and that the amine transmitters are presumed to be removed largely by diffusion back to their point of origin followed by active re-uptake into the nerve terminal. From any point of view, then, receptor-transmitter combinations are unlikely to exist in easily detectable quantities, and they may be unstable after isolation.

The formation of receptor-transmitter combinations at a postsynaptic membrane leads, within as little as half a millisecond, to a change in electrical potential across the membrane. The result, referred to as a postsynaptic potential, is caused by changes in membrane permeability to one or more ions; an increase in permeability to Na^+ reduces the negative potential (depolarization), while an increase in permeability to K^+ or Cl^- leads to hyperpolarization. These changes in membrane potential persist at least as long as the transmitter-receptor combination is intact. If, before decay of the postsynaptic potential occurs, another quantal release of transmitter takes place, the overall effect is additive in an algebraic sense. Thus the magnitude of the postsynaptic potential depends upon the frequency of arriving impulses as well as upon the quantity and kind of transmitter that is released by each impulse. Where depolarizing potentials are involved, the electrical charge eventually spreads from the dendrites through the cell body to the axon hillock. Since this region is electrically excitable a depolarizing potential of sufficient magnitude will initiate an action potential. The action potential not only travels down the axon but may also be reflected back into the cell body, with the probable result that the postsynaptic potential is in effect erased, leaving the dendrites and cell body free to respond freshly to another set of arriving impulses.

Since a depolarizing potential may ultimately lead to an action potential it is referred to as an excitatory postsynaptic potential (EPSP); in contrast hyperpolarization moves the cell potential away from the point at which it may produce an action potential and it therefore is referred to as an inhibitory postsynaptic potential (IPSP). Just as PSPs may sum at one particular synapse in response to a sequence of arriving impulses (temporal summation) so also may they sum throughout a cell body in response to impulses arriving at many synapses. Such spatial summation may involve adding the positive effect of an EPSP to the negative effect of an IPSP. Whether or not the cell produces an action potential depends upon whether EPSPs outweigh IPSPs.

All of these effects depend upon graded changes in membrane permeability to Na^+, K^+, or Cl^-. Transmitters such as glycine and gamma aminobutyric acid are believed to be responsible for IPSPs, noradrenalin is considered to produce EPSPs, while other transmitters may be excitatory or inhibitory, depending upon the structure of the membrane upon which they impinge. The exact mechanism by which transmitters alter permeability of the postsynaptic membrane is still unknown. There are in general two kinds of hypotheses. One considers that the transmitter combines with a membrane-bound protein receptor in such a way as to alter the configuration of the protein, and hence of the membrane, directly, while the other regards the transmitter as a trigger that sets off a sequence of biochemical events which ultimately leads to a reversible change in membrane permeability.

The prostaglandins, a class of substances that are found throughout the body, are implicated in some way in neuronal membrane function. It appears that they may be synthesized from membrane-bound phospholipids in direct response to arriving nerve impulses. Since a conversion of one membrane substance to another necessarily involves some kind of a change in membrane structure and since it is presumed that changes in membrane structure are the prerequisites for permeability changes, it is possible that the prostaglandins may be involved in the response of the postsynaptic membrane. More specific details await further research.

If, as seems likely, the proper functioning of the postsynaptic membrane requires a closely timed sequence of transmitter-receptor combination and separation, any agent that would alter the time course of the reaction would have a profound effect upon the information-processing function of the brain. It is believed that some chemical therapeutic agents may alter the responsiveness of the postsynaptic membrane and that some other drugs may function as "false transmitters," in the sense that their combinations with receptors might last so long as to block normal responsiveness to naturally occurring transmitters. Finally, it is conceivable that some disease states might be caused by synthesis, within the brain, of false transmitters.

9

Memory Storage and Retrieval

A SEQUENCE OF numbers, such as 867—9143, is written on a card and presented to a cooperating subject. Just before presentation he is told that he will be shown the card for only 10 seconds and asked to reproduce the sequence several minutes later. He is then shown another group of numbers and given similar instructions modified by the additional information that it represents his new telephone number. In each instance he will probably repeat the sequence to himself several times until he learns it, and he will be able to repeat it on demand soon after. In the second instance he will probably also be able to repeat the sequence several days later. The ability to acquire information and retrieve it at some future time is familiar to all of us. If the information is retrievable at least some aspects of it must have been stored. By "memory" we mean storage of information. Learning, which is taken as equivalent to the acquisition process, will be discussed in the following chapter.

A more detailed look at the neural processes will be helpful. The card containing the number sequence produced an image upon the eye, whose ganglion cells were then stimulated to initiate trains of impulses. The impulse flow traveled along selected fibers of the optic nerve, through the optic chiasma, where most of the fibers cross to the opposite side, and finally to a neural relay station known as the lateral geniculate nucleus, located in the thalamic region. At this location the target neurons are probably modified by a wide range of ongoing neural signals from other parts of the brain. They "fire" in response to the mixture of new and ongoing information, and their fibers project to neurons at the rear of the skull, the so-called optic cortex. These in turn produce trains of impulses which flow to other regions of the brain.

The numbers on the card, representing specific information, were encoded into trains of precisely patterned impulses. For the moment at least the information on the card was expressed as patterns of neural activity. Does the retention of the information require that these patterns persist forever after or are there ways in which they can be further encoded into structural changes in the brain? It has been pointed out in Chapter 7 that a reverberating circuit will occur when certain threshold requirements are met and that such a circuit constitutes a memory. Many years ago it was supposed that most, if not all, memory in the brain was achieved by means of reverberating circuits. More recently researchers have leaned toward the view that structural alterations in the brain are required for information storage. Although reverberating circuits fell from favor because there does not seem to be enough of them available to store the required information, some of the present hypotheses suffer from the same defect. It will be useful, then, to review the boundary conditions, that is, the total information storage required, the conceivable locations of such storage, and the rules that determine the storage process. First, however, it will be profitable to review the results of an early experimental approach to the problem.

It is relatively easy to observe learning in small experimental animals under well-defined conditions. A rat will be allowed to wander through a maze until it reaches a location at which food is placed. If hungry it will be motivated by the reward to return to the goal as rapidly as possible after having been repositioned at the starting point. The time required and the number of errors (turns into blind alleys) decrease with successive trials. The animal learns the correct path and will then perform relatively reproducibly. If it is then returned to its home cage and again placed at the starting point of the maze several days later, it will exhibit only a little hesitancy in attaining the goal. Clearly, information about the learned task has been stored somewhere.

In an attempt to find out where the memory might be located specific small regions were severed or removed from the brains of a group of rats in which such memory had already been demonstrated. The rationale for this approach followed from the generally successful studies of many neuroanatomists who were able to localize other brain functions by this technique. It was a matter of considerable surprise to learn that the memory of the task could not be interfered with by removal of any small region. Removal of much larger regions impaired general performance but again there was no indication of localization of memory.

Although it might have been concluded that the memory for this task did not reside in the brain at all, it seemed more reasonable to conclude that the memory was stored redundantly in many regions of the brain. Much subsequent experience has led to the view that portions of the remembered task are stored in widely scattered sites throughout the brain. There may be many copies of each portion.

Thus the stored information, or the memory engram as it is sometimes called, is not to be conceived of as similar to a section of a photograph, or a length of magnetic tape, where all the relevant information is precisely organized. Rather it is better represented as an interconnected array of fragments of information from which the complete memory has to be reconstructed upon each demand. This concept is reminiscent of the reliable net of subgroups of imperfect cells outlined in Chapter 7 (page 95).

Redundancy and fragmentation are thus likely to be among the boundary conditions. Another important condition has to do with the quantity of information stored. It has already been mentioned (Chapter 7) that, of the various estimates made, the calculation of 10^{20} bits of information stored during a lifetime appears to be the most reasonable. This must mean that, if the

patterns of neural impulses are encoded into structural alterations, there should be 10^{20} sites at which such alterations can
occur. Much consideration has been given to the synapse as the
site of memory storage, and it has been suggested that the actual
record consists of an irreversible alteration in the responsivity of
the synapse. However, there are about 10 billion neurons and, if
each has an average of 1,000 synaptic junctions, there are only 10^{13}
synapses available for all brain function, that is, 1 ten-millionth of
the number needed for single copies of the lifetime information
storage. Clearly, the unit of storage must have dimensions very
much smaller than that of the synapse. Considerations such as these
lead to the view that information is stored in units of molecular
dimensions.

Molecular storage of biological information is not a new
concept. For many years it has been recognized that all of the
minutely detailed information transmitted from one generation to
the next is encoded in DNA molecules. The code operates as
follows. Individual members in a sequence of deoxyribonucleo-
tides in DNA differ from each other with respect to the identity
of the purine or pyrimidine bases (adenine, guanine, thymine, and
cytosine) which they contain. Each sequence of three nucleotides, containing specific bases, constitutes a "word" of genetic
information in the sense that it ultimately specifies the selection of
a particular amino acid at a particular location when a protein
molecule is synthesized. DNA is thought of as a permanent
residue of genetic information, that is, as a genetic "memory."
The readout from the memory occurs when a "derepressor"
molecule dislodges a "repressor" molecule from a special section
of the DNA known as an operator. An adjacent section, the
operon, then directs the synthesis of RNA, which differs from
DNA both with respect to the pentose sugar (RNA has ribose
while DNA has desoxyribose) and with respect to the sequence of
bases (guanine and cytosine are interchanged, while thymine in
DNA is replaced by uracil in RNA). Thus, a "base-paired,"
biologically impermanent transcription of the DNA molecule is
accomplished. While it exists this newly synthesized RNA then
directs the synthesis of a specific protein.

Molecular storage of information, whether in DNA or in any
other large molecule, ultimately depends upon the sequences of

the functional groups. In DNA each group of three nucleotides constitutes one functional group; in proteins we may reasonably suppose that each amino acid constitutes a functional group. Without prejudging the question, let us assume for the moment that memory of neural events is ultimately stored in a peptide which contains one of each of the 20 most common amino acids. The number of distinct peptides will be equal to the number of permutations of 20 amino acids, which is 2.4×10^{18} . We now need to know the minimum number of bits that would be required to specify each peptide. Since one amino acid from the list of 20 must be selected for each position, a five-bit number is needed at each location, and 20 such numbers are required for the whole chain. Thus 100 bits of information will specify the whole chain, and each specific peptide is the equivalent to, and can store, 100 bits of information. All possible permutations of the hypothetical 20-amino-acid peptide are thus capable of storing $100 \times 2.4 \times 10^{28} = 2.4 \times 10^{20}$ bits of information, a number that approximates the estimated lifetime storage. If the peptide were only twice as large, containing two of each amino acid, the information content would be raised to the power of 2, giving the number 5.76 $\times 10^{40}$—more than enough to account for extensive redundancy of the lifetime information.

Thus quantity and redundancy, two important boundary conditions, are easily accounted for by molecular storage of neural information. Another boundary condition concerns the physical space required to store so many individual molecules. Will their total weight be so great as to make storage impossible? Returning to the 2.4×10^{18} individual variants (molecules) of the hypothetical 20-amino-acid peptide, it can be calculated by dividing by Avogodro's number (the number of molecules in a mole) that there are $2.4 \times 10^{18}/6 \times 10^{23} = 4 \times 10^{6}$ moles of the peptide, whose molecular weight would be about 2,500. Thus the sum of all variants of the peptide would weigh $2,500 \times 4 \times 10^{6} = 10^{2}$ grams. This amount of peptide, or its equivalent if combined into larger peptides or proteins, could be contained in 2×10^{6} neurons having an average weight of 5×10^{8} grams and an average protein content of 10%. If redundancy required an average of 10^{3} copies of such memory molecules, then 2×10^{9} neurons, or about 15% of the available number, would be required. Alternatively, it could be stated that 15% of the protein in each neuron would ultimately be needed for memory storage. Thus another important boundary condition is met; there is enough physical space to store redundant information in this form, even if information storage occurs exclusively in neurons and not at all in glial cells.

There are important boundary conditions relating to speed of storage and speed of readout. The initial information input is first encoded into trains of neural impulses; these pass rapidly along axons and produce electrical field changes at synaptic junctions that may last for only a few milliseconds. If further encoding into molecular synthesis or reorganization is to occur, the unitary chemical changes would have to take place within that short time interval. That is, a specific pattern of impulses may pass repetitively (reverberate) over a given synapse, but it is necessary that with each pass at least one lasting chemical event, such as the mobilization of one amino acid, should occur, if there is to be ultimate translation of neural patterns into chemical synthesis. The boundary question, then, is this: can the necessary chemical events occur within a few milliseconds? A partial answer to this question can be obtained by considering the fastest known rates of enzyme synthesis, which approximate 10^6 moles of product synthesized each minute by a mole of enzyme. Converting to a single molecule basis, the fastest enzymes can direct the synthesis of $10^6/60 \times 10^3 = 16$ molecules per millisecond. Thus chemical synthesis can occur at the required rate. What is unknown, of course, is whether synthesis directed by neural impulses can occur at rates comparable to enzyme synthesis. Enzymes facilitate chemical reaction by combining with substrate molecules to form reaction complexes. It could be hypothesized that the consequences of patterns of impulses at the postsynaptic location are the production of very small regions of highly organized electrical fields and that such regions would be analogous, in their specificity, to those portions of an enzyme molecule that combine with substrate molecules. Whether this or other speculations have any validity is a question for future research to determine.

The last boundary condition concerns readout. Assume that the sense of the foregoing discussion approximates reality. Then the rapidly flowing neural impulses have been encoded, by chemical synthesis, into specific molecules which can store the information after the impulse flow dies out. What is required now is a means of regenerating specific trains of impulses from these molecules, rapidly but only upon demand. To postulate that the "memory molecules" permanently change synaptic transmisssion is of little help for, as previously mentioned, there are about 10^{-7} of the needed number of "memory" synapses. Furthermore, the "only upon demand" clause of the boundary condition is not met by such a postulate, since a permanently altered synapse ought to be responsive all of the time to many nonspecific inputs. Up to the present time this aspect of the problem of memory has not received much attention.

Some Hypothetical Memory Molecules

Memory usually implies a more or less permanent storage of information. If an individual molecule is to be a storage site, it should either be resistant to biochemical alteration or capable of continued replicaton. Since DNA is among the most stable molecular species known, capable of preserving genetic information over a lifetime, it was natural to look to the DNA-RNA system as a possible source of molecular storage of neural information.

The first efforts in this direction implicated RNA directly, when it was observed that the chemical composition of RNA changed after a learning trial; the RNA obtained from the neuronal nuclei of rat brain contained an increased proportion of the purine base adenine to the pyrimidine base cytosine. It was postulated that new RNA molecules were synthesized directly under the influence of the patterned neuronal impulses and that subsequently the synthesis of a specific protein was directed by the new RNA. It was further suggested that it was the specific protein that functioned as the repository of the information and the retrieval consisted in the breakdown of the protein in response to other neural signals. The breakdown products were postulated to influence the release of transmitters which then excited the postsynaptic neuron. Since this hypothesis requires the breakdown of the protein when it is utilized for retrieval of memory, permanence of memory requires that a replenishment occur, presumably still under the influence of the specific RNA, and that the RNA should therefore be a very durable molecule. However, from what is known of RNA metabolism this is unlikely; RNA decays at a much faster rate than does memory.

Another hypothesis utilizes the mechanism of the genetic code. It is postulated that the patterned neural impulse activates specific derepressor molecules which allow the operator region of the DNA molecule to initiate specific RNA synthesis by the operon region. The memory-specific RNA is in turn postulated to direct the synthesis of a memory-specific protein. The proponents of this hypothesis suggest that the protein then produces a permanent facilitated synaptic pathway, which represent the memory. As has been pointed out above, such hypotheses require extravagant use of synapses; there are about 10^{-7} as many synapses as needed for the purpose.

Aside from peptides, proteins, and RNA, little or no attention has been given to other molecular species as possible repositories of information, largely on the grounds that sufficient complexity is lacking in smaller molecules and also on the assumption that they are likely to be less permanent. The requirement for permanence of the individual molecule is not absolute; any neurochemical feedback system that results in resynthesis of exact copies of the "memory molecule" would serve the purpose.

The assumption that, if memory is encoded into a molecule, it can only be a single large molecule whose informative sections are linked by covalent bonds appears so reasonable upon first presentation that alternatives are never considered. However, the characteristics of such a large molecule could be simulated by juxtaposition of many smaller molecules provided that their location relative to each other were somehow fixed. Once the problem is stated in this manner other possibilities become apparent. For example, it has been pointed out (Chapter 3) that the concentrations of cerebrosides and cerebroside sulfates change only slightly throughout life and that each of these lipid classes is composed of individual members differing with respect to their individual fatty acids, of which there are at least 28 varieties. Thus a row of 20 cerebroside molecules, if considered as a unit of storage, could store as much information as a 20-

amino-acid peptide. Since such storage would occur predominantly in the myelin that envelops the axon, a memory hypothesis employing cerebrosides would have to postulate that readout occurs not at synaptic junctions but along the axon as it is traversed by the neural impulse. Readout of the information might then consist in the modification of a train of impulses by interaction with cerebrosides whose location is crucial to further propagation of the impulse—perhaps those located near the nodes of Ranvier.

The evidence for molecular storage of information is presently based upon two lines of investigation. The first is directed at a detailed study of procedures which interfere with memory or its retrieval; the second involves a controversial field of study designated as "chemical transfer of memory."

The detailed study of interference with memory overlaps considerably with the subject of the following chapter; only a brief outline will be presented here. It has been recognized for many years that memory phenomena may be divided into at least two classes: short- and long-term memory. Although the definition of "short-term memory" varies from a few seconds to a few hours according to the particular experimental conditions employed, it is agreed without exception that memory persisting beyond a week has a different basis. The process of acquiring long-term memory is known as consolidation, and some of the factors known to interfere with it offer considerable support for the molecular hypothesis.

The phenomenom of retrograde amnesia following a concussion or another kind of head injury was described 100 years ago. The loss of memory is most severe for recent events. The experimental study of retrograde amnesia was facilitated by the observation that there is an apparent loss of memory for recent events following the therapeutic use of electroconvulsive shock (ECS). Subsequently, detailed experiments were extended to animals who had learned specific performance tasks. In some instances spontaneous recovery of memory occurred after ECS; in others the shock appeared to be received by the subjects as if it were a learned stimulus that governed future response. There is general agreement, however, that ECS can produce retrograde amnesia under carefully controlled conditions. Other conditions and agents that have been reported to lead to retrograde amnesia include anoxia, large temperature change, anaesthesia, increased carbon dioxide intake, specific brain injury, and administration of several kinds of antibiotics. This last group constitutes a widely used tool for exploration of the chemical basis of memory because these substances inhibit synthesis of RNA or protein.

One problem with such substances, which are usually injected directly into the brains of experimental animals, is that general toxicity and other side effects confuse the interpretation of the results. However, one inhibitor of cerebral protein synthesis, acetoxycycloheximide, is extremely potent as an inhibitor at doses which produce minimal side effects. When this substance is injected 5 minutes before training the animals learn as well as controls injected with sodium chloride solution and remember the learned tasks 3 hours later. However, when tested for retention at times ranging from 6 hours to 6 weeks later, they remembered much less effectively than did the controls. Since protein synthesis was almost completely inhibited at the time training occurred as well as during the test 3 hours later, it was concluded that learning and short-term memory were not critically dependent upon protein synthesis but that long-term memory could not occur without associated protein synthesis.

The conclusion that protein synthesis is required for establishment of long-term memory is likely to be the furthest one can go with this approach. No doubt further research will show the subcellular and anatomical localization of the required protein synthesis, and it may even be possible to define and chemically characterize some specific proteins. However, unless such efforts succeed in demonstrating that only a specific protein, and no other substance, need be interfered with in order to prevent long-term memory, it will still remain as a possibility that the protein only mediates information storage, either in some other molecules or by producing some localized anatomical changes.

Direct demonstration that memory resides in protein or peptide molecules would seem to be almost impossible to achieve. Yet that is precisely the goal of the "memory transfer" experiments.

Interanimal Transfer of Memory?

The reasoning was as follows. Teach an animal to perform a simple task. If its memory of that task is encoded in the specific structure of some complex molecules then perhaps those molecules can be removed from its brain and injected into a recipient animal where they might conceivably relocate in the appropriate brain region. If all of this has occured then it should be possible to demonstrate that the recipient animal knows the task without undergoing a learning experience. Positive results, in addition to challenging many concepts of neural organization and the exclusivity of the blood-brain barrier, would be clear evidence for the existence of memory molecules.

Although these results have not yet, and may never be, attained, the history of the experimentation to date has produced some useful knowledge, as well as a degree of controversy that seldom occurs in science. The earliest studies, which began with a species of flatworm known as Planaria, are still encumbered by serious questions concerning the extent of learning and conditioning that can be reproducibly observed in these worms. The early reports claimed that, when a planarian whose progress through a maze had apparently been learned was ground up and fed to another planarian, the second worm required fewer trials than the first to traverse the maze. The possibility that the improved performance was due to transfer of memory almost immediately led to other experiments employing mice and rats as the experimental subjects. The tasks that were learned were not different from those employed in more conservative studies of learning and memory, but at the conclusion of the learning period the brains were removed from the trained animals and either a portion of the whole brain or a specific extract was injected into untrained recipients, who then appeared to "know" the required task without learning it. By such techniques "transfer of memory" was reported in a variety of investigations by seven different groups of researchers while many other laboratories reported failure to reproduce the results. The learned tasks in the successful experiments included: approach to a food cup conditioned by a stimulus of light or sound; selection of either the lighted or dark branch of a T-maze; and time required to escape from a given location after presentation of a cue. In most cases the trained animals learned as a result of a positive reinforcement (food) or a negative reinforcement (foot shock) while the recipient animals were not reinforced. The transferred material varied between experiments from homogenates of whole brain in some to RNA extracts in others and partially purified peptide extracts in still other experiments. It will be useful to consider two examples.

The first experiment to be discussed deals with observations of the rate of learning of recipient rats that were given RNA obtained from the brains of donors that had been trained according to the following experimenal paradigm. A large cage was equipped with a bar-press lever on one side and a device for dispensing small quantities of sweetened milk on the other side. The dispenser could be held in the delivery position for any chosen time interval and could be operated either by the animal pressing the bar or by the experimenter externally. In order to obtain milk the animal would have to learn to press the bar, then cross the cage, and lick the milk during the 5 to 10 seconds that the dispenser remained in the up position. This is apparently a difficult task and most of the animals do not obtain milk readily under such circumstances unless they have learned the task in two steps. The first step consists in learning that milk is present at the dispenser and that the dispenser will move to the delivery position only when preceded by a loud click. After learning this part of the task, which is accomplished by randomly presenting the click followed by the reward (milk), the learning proceeds to the next stage, where the dispenser is in the nondelivery position and no click occurs unless the rat happens to press the bar. The bar presses are initially random but, since each is always followed by a click and presentation of the reward, the rat rapidly learns the second stage, during which a barpress that occurs only while the dispenser is down will raise it to the delivery position for 20 seconds. A bar press during the 20 seconds that the dispenser is up does not result in the presentation of an additional quantity of milk. It was reasoned that, if the learning experience is encoded in molecular form, injection of the appropriate molecules obtained from the donor brain into the cerebrospinal fluid of the recipients would make it possible for the recipients to perform the second stage (the required bar pressing) without having to be taught the first stage (the association of the click with the food reward).

RNA was obtained from donor brains, some from animals that had learned the complete task and some from controls that had never been in the learning environment. In each case a portion of the RNA was set aside while another portion was subjected to the action of the enzyme ribonuclease, which broke it down to a less organized structure. After 5 days of testing, only those recipients who had received intact RNA from trained donors were able to perform the task reliably. It seemed to be a valid conclusion, from these and other experiments by this research group, that the ability to learn the task was increased specifically as a result of injection of intact RNA from trained donors. However, it is difficult to know exactly what was transferred—specific information about the task itself or a greatly increased alertness to the test conditions which would improve the rate of learning in the RNA recipients.

Another experimental paradigm employed shock-avoidance conditioning to train donor rats. They were allowed to move freely for 3 minutes between the light and dark chambers of a two-chamber container. Their normal preference was to spend more than half of the time in the dark chamber. Subsequently, entry into the dark chamber was accompanied by an electric shock which caused the rats to learn to avoid the dark chamber. The brains were removed and extracted to obtain a concentrate of a peptide. The material was then injected into the brains of recipient mice. If the peptide concentrate was derived from trained donors, the recipient mice then spent much more time in the lighted chamber than they did prior to the injection. Extracts from control (untrained) donors were without effect. Furthermore, if the peptide concentrate from trained donors was first subjected to the action of the enzyme trypsin (which breaks down the chemical bonds between amino acids in peptides and proteins), injection was then without effect on the recipients.

The peptide was analyzed to determine its chemical structure and found to contain 15 amino acids. It was synthesized chemically and concentrates of varying purity were provided to two other researchers. Injection of the synthetic material, scoto-phobin, into mice also resulted in avoidance of the dark chamber, just as in the "memory transfer" experiments.

Initially researchers in the field thought that they had a tool by which to study the molecular coding of specific information. That tool, as discussed above, was the "memory transfer" experiment. Because the concept of memory transfer seemed so out of place with a large body of information about the highly specific **organization of the central nervous system, as well as the diffi**-culty in reproducing results, many scientists were highly critical of this field of study. At the present time the region of disagree-ment seems to have contracted somewhat; the proponents have recognized the experimental pitfalls and the overinterpretations of the earlier results, while at least some of the critics, having accepted the experimental validity of some of the later results, have focused on alternate explanations. It is suggested that the extracted substances have the properties of general activators of behavior and that the more alert or more active recipients will perform better and thus appear to demonstrate "transferred memory." On the other hand, fewer of the proponents now talk about memory transfer. Instead, the recipients are thought to have undergone behavioral modification as a result of the injec-tion of the specific extract. However, whether activation, behav-ioral modification, or something in between is occurring, it does seem as of this writing that in at least some of the experiments the transferred extract has been produced in the donor brain in response to the initial learning trials. This in itself would be an important conclusion and well worth the effort because it would clearly indicate that the process of learning and perhaps consoli-dation of memory as well may require specific endogenous chemical entities that can be produced upon demand. Whether such substances would in any instances function as "memory molecules" would depend upon the degree of specificity of the information they might contain.

Retrieval of Stored Information

If the information contained in a pattern of neural impulses is encoded into specific memory molecules for long-term storage and if the information-processing function of the brain is accomplished via trains of ongoing neural impulses, then there must be a way to reconstruct the neural patterns from the stored molecules. Many of the experiments designed to explore the chemical basis of long-term memory employ inhibitors of RNA or protein synthesis. In all such cases the experimenter must respond to the alternate interpretation that the inhibitor has interfered with the expression of memory (retrieval) rather than with memory itself. When the inability to demonstrate memory lasts well beyond the period during which the inhibitor is effective, it is considered good evidence that storage has been blocked.

In some experiments, however, there appears to be a gradual recovery of memory. In such cases it is a reasonable conclusion that the inhibitor is somehow involved in the retrieval process. The following account of an experiment appears to be a particularly informative example of interference with retrieval, although the authors chose a different interpretation. The experimental animals were homing salmon. Their characteristic and renowned behavior, the ability to find their way over long distances to "home" waters, apparently depends upon a long-term memory. It has been found that an increase in the electrical activity of the olfactory bulb of the brain occurs when various waters are infused through the nostrils of these animals. In particular, more activity is produced by home water than by water obtained from similar pools that were never inhabited by the particular subjects. Thus activation correlated with memory of the home water can presumably be observed as an electrophysiological response in the olfactory bulb. When either RNA or protein synthesis inhibitors are injected into the brain, the electrophysiological response to pond water diminishes and the difference between responses to home and other waters disappears for 4 to 7 hours after the injection. Recovery of the response occurs within the next 20 hours. Since it seems most reasonable to regard the differential electrophysiological response as at least a partial expression of a naturally acquired memory, these experiments strongly implicate RNA and protein in the expression (retrieval) of memory. That is, retrieval of a well-stored memory cannot occur unless accompanied by concurrent synthesis of RNA and protein.

Other experiments which appear to show recovery of

memory long after an injection of an inhibitor of RNA or protein synthesis are confounded by an experimental design which seeks to assess memory by measuring a factor designated as "savings." An animal is trained (learns) to respond to a behavioral task by demonstrating a certain proportion of correct responses; for example, the animal learns to choose the lighted area of a branched pathway (a "Y" maze) 9 out of 10 times, when the light is randomly varied from one branch to the other. Its memory is then tested in the same trial situation, and savings are calculated from the proportion of errors in each instance. For example, if during the learning phase 12 series of trials were required before the desired performance of 9 out of 10 trials was attained and during the memory retest phase 3 series of trials were required, the savings would be calculated as $100 \times (12 - 3)/12 = 75\%$. The experimental design therefore measures the efficiency of relearning. It is assumed that a greater efficiency is related to some degree of memory for the task. When inhibitors reduce savings it is assumed that either the long-term memory was disrupted or that an interference with retrieval occurred. Recently it has been reported that inhibitors previously thought to disrupt storage may instead have disrupted retrieval. One research group found that, having injected a protein synthesis inhibitor a few minutes after training, the apparent memory deficit 5 days later could be reversed by an injection of NaCl into the brain of the experimental animals and that, if other cations (K^+, Li^+, Ca^{++}, or Mg^{++}) were injected along with the inhibitor, the memory deficit never appeared. Another research group found a spontaneous recovery when animals were retested several days after having received an injection of a protein synthesis inhibitor just prior to training. These researchers present a plausible explanation of the recovery of memory observed by several research groups. They suggest that memory is maintained only by a continued resynthesis of the specific molecules in which the information is stored, that a certain minimum number of memory molecules are required to allow retrieval, and that the increase in the total number constitutes the long-term storage process. Appearance of memory on retesting would then depend on how many memory molecules were produced by the initial training and on how extensively their amplified resynthesis was interfered with by the inhibitors.

An equally plausible explanation focuses on the experimental design of the savings experiment. When savings are less than 100%, what is actually observed is a relearning process. Although it may depend on prior memory, it may also depend on conditions governing the observation of savings. That is, the inhibitor may interfere with the learning process as a consequence of its long-term effect on neurochemical structure. Recovery of memory, which sometimes has been reported after ECS, has been shown to depend upon the opportunity for relearning during repeated retesting. No recovery occurred if relearning was excluded from the experimental design. Similar effects are likely to contribute to the recovery observed with protein synthesis inhibitors.

Thus relearning, memory storage, and retrieval are dependent in various ways upon synthesis of macromolecules such as RNA or proteins. The following chapter will examine the details of the learning phase with respect to correlated neurochemical events.

10

Chemical Correlates of Learning

THE DESIGN OF experimental studies of learning is crucial because it is desirable to study the initial acquisition process separated as far as possible from the storage process. Since demonstrations that learning has occurred are carried out some time after the learning process, and thus depend upon memory of the learned event, it would seem that the problems involved in differentiating learning from memory are semantic rather than biological. A way out of the impasse has been sought by recourse to the concepts of short- and long-term memory. Thus permanent storage is taken as equivalent to memory whereas transient storage is part, but not all, of the learning process.

Learning, then, must require the temporary storage of information while it is being further processed and evaluated, that is, while "insight" develops. Long-term storage may include the primary information (as in the example of simple recall which introduced Chapter 9) but it must necessarily include any insight derived during the learning experience. That is, if a rat is exposed to a flash of light a few seconds before receiving an electric shock and eventually learns to run to a safe area as soon as the light flashes, its remembrance of the escape procedure weeks later implies that the stimuli of being picked up and placed in the recognizable test cage will alert it to seek escape when the light flashes. What is stored in long-term memory is the rat equivalent of "handling plus this cage plus that light means danger." Some of the individual events of the training trial may also be stored, but we would not expect a rapid expression of insight unless the rat's conclusions about these events had also been stored.

We can therefore semantically and biologically separate learning from memory; the retention (which may be short- or long-term) of the individual events in the training process is required to form the insight, which should then be stored in long-term memory. What is needed, then, is an experiment that will measure the chemical correlates of the insight process. Before considering the details and results of such an experiment it will be useful to examine some earlier approaches to the problem.

These derive from the initial attempts to identify short-term memory. The general concept of different modes of memory arose from two separate fields of research and led to two different estimates of the duration of short-term memory. Psychological studies of learning and memory indicated that an interference with remembering could be demonstrated to occur within seconds of the initial learning experience, from which it was concluded that repetition of primary patterns of neural activity could be considered as equivalent to the short-term phase. On the other hand, interference with associated neuro-chemical events by means of inhibitors indicated that consolidation of memory required many days, while adequate memory could be demonstrated at least several hours after injection of the inhibitor. Thus if memory was to be separated into short- and long-term phases, the time span of the short-term phase, by these procedures, seemed to range from minutes to hours. It was obvious to bridge these two estimates by postulating an inter-mediate-term memory phase. Figure 10-1 schematically represents the time sequence of the three phases. Learning would certainly require the existence of the first phase and could easily overlap to include part or all of the second phase. However, there is some reason to believe that learning might continue to occur for

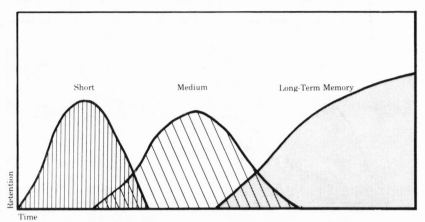

Figure 10-1. A sequential model of memory. Information first acquired in short-term memory is then stored in medium-term memory and, from there, in long-term memory.

several days. The usual procedure to test for the occurrence of learning and memory first firmly establishes the required performance by extensive training of an experimental animal; it then proceeds to retest the same animal successively over a period of hours, days, and weeks. Under these conditions the memory appears to be fairly constant—that is, it seems as if all learning has occurred during the initial training period. However, when the training is less extensive, so that the animals do not learn completely during the first training session, it is found that if separate subgroups are tested, not repetitively but only once more at varying times after the training, quite different results are obtained. There seems to be a period of several days during which the number of trials required to reach the performance criterion are relatively constant, but at some later time the required number of trials drops considerably. Four points are important. First, these observations seem to be a clear-cut demonstration of memory; a learning trial experienced at a certain time has influenced subsequent performance only after many days, presumably when the results of that learning became available for the first time, to augment further learning. Second, it seems that learning can draw not only on the substrate of short-term memory (which presumably involves recurrent neural responses to the

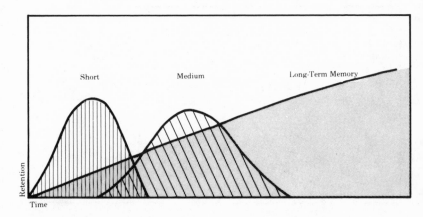

Figure 10-2. A parallel model of memory. Information is stored in short-term memory and then transferred to medium-term memory. At the same time, consolidation into long-term memory begins by a parallel path which does not involve transfer from short- or medium-term memory.

initial information input), but it also utilizes the consolidated long-term memory store. Third, there is a transition phase of a few days, during which the initial experience, even though it is in the process of being recorded in long-term memory, is not available for recall to augment learning. And fourth, when the delay between the training and testing extended beyond 2 weeks, the long-term store of the initial experience was no longer retrievable. That is, the experience appears to have been forgotten.

To recapitulate, it appears that learning can be augmented by interaction with short-term and long-term memory, but not with intermediate-term memory. The precise number of hours and days involved in these processes should not be regarded as rigidly fixed; the times probably depend upon the nature of the task and the extent of under- or overtraining. However, the sequence of phenomena is reproducible. Thus there are at least two times when learning might be studied; one is associated with the initial neural input and the other occurs after the requisite degree of consolidation has been obtained.

Rapid Neurochemical Changes Associated with Learning

Direct observation of neurochemical changes that might occur with the short-term retention of the primary neural input is exceedingly difficult and has not yet been attempted, but it has been possible to study the changes that take place less than an hour after a brief learning experience.

A particularly informative experiment was carried out as follows. A cage with a wire grid floor was divided into two sections. One section had an escape platform so that when the mouse within it received electric shock through the floor it was able to jump onto the platform. The other section had no such escape. A pair of mice was placed in the cage, the experimental mouse in the section with the escape platform and the control in the section without an escape. A centrally located light and buzzer signaled the advent of a shock for 3 seconds. Both mice received the shock simultaneously, for equal lengths of time, until the experimental mouse jumped to the escape platform. After escaping from the shock the experimental mouse was returned to the grid floor and the sequence of signal, shock, and escape was repeated. After a few trials the experimental mouse learned to jump to the platform as soon as the signal appeared, thus avoiding the shock. Under these conditions the control mouse did not receive the shock either. By 10 minutes the test mouse had learned to avoid the shock 9 out of 10 times. After another 5 minutes of training the brains of the two mice were removed. Half an hour prior to the initiation of the training each mouse had been injected with a radioactive tracer substance so that neurochemical changes could be followed. In this particular experiment the labeled molecule was the nucleoside uridine—the molecule formed by combining uracil with ribose.

When the brains of a large number of such yoked pairs of experimental and control mice were analyzed the following differences were consistently observed. The amount of label incorporated into RNA obtained from either the cell nuclei or the ribosomal fraction of the entire brain was much greater for the experimental than for the control animals. When particular brain regions were studied it was found that the increase was characteristic of limbic system structures. In contrast, incorporation of label into RNA obtained from the outer layers of the cortex was decreased in the experimental group compared to the controls. These effects were specific to the brain; there were no differences between experimental and control animals in incorporation of label into RNA derived from the liver or kidney. The labeled RNA was heterogeneous—the tracer uridine could be found in all molecular species of RNA. Thus there is no evidence from these experiments for a special molecular form of RNA associated with learning.

The experimenters sought to define more closely the particular aspect of the learning experience that was associated with the increased incorporation of label into RNA. The direct effect of shock was eliminated since each yoked control received the same amount of shock as its experimental counterpart. Moreover, the yoked controls did not incorporate more label into RNA than did randomly shocked mice or mice allowed to rest quietly in their cages. Thus any nonspecific stimuli associated with the training was eliminated. The possibility that the increased incorporation occurred during the time period after learning had been established was eliminated by first training the mice and then injecting the radioactive uridine. These animals did not show increased incorporation of label into RNA. Thus there was a strong inference that neither random stimuli nor performance after learning could be associated with the observed results and that it was during the learning (insight) phase that the increased incorporation occurred.

To confirm the inference the learning experiment was run backwards. If an animal, which has learned to associate a conditioned stimulus (light or sound) with an unconditioned stimulus (electric shock), is then repeatedly exposed to the conditioned stimulus but never to the unconditioned stimulus, it will eventually "unlearn" the association. That is, a new insight will develop, signifying that the light and buzzer are no longer a portent of danger. Under such conditions the response to the buzzer (in this case, jumping onto the escape shelf) will gradually disappear. This process, known as "extinction," was applied to a group of mice which had received an injection of radioactive uridine after training but prior to extinction. Once again there was an increased incorporation of label into RNA. Once again the inference was strong that the observed results occurred during the insight phase, since it had already been shown that increased incorporation of label did not occur if the mice were injected after training, and it was unlikely that the final phase of extinction, in which the mice did not respond at all, should be associated with any neuro-chemical differences.

The same group of experimenters subsequently carried out a study on the incorporation of radioactive phosphate into a protein fraction isolated from neuronal nuclei. Once again there was an increase in incorporation of label into the protein derived from the trained animal when compared to yoked controls or to randomly shocked animals. The increase in the phosphate label was due entirely to an increase in phosphoserine. Radioactivity of a similar phosphorylated amino acid, phosphothreonine, was not different between the experimental and control groups. Again limbic system structures were implicated in the increased incor-poration of label. However, it was found that, when rats were trained for 6 successive days and then injected and trained again on the 7th day, there was an increase in the incorporation of labeled phosphate. These results contrasted with those for uridine incorporation, in which it was found that the increased incor-poration of label was apparently associated with the insight phase. The researchers surmised that a "reminding," rather than an insight, phenomenon was associated with the results. How-ever, in these experiments the 5-minute training period probably produced incomplete learning since the average response of the first day was 6 out of 10 trials. It is possible that additional learning was associated with long-term memory (see discussion of Figure 10-2) existing during the 7th day of these experiments and that the insight hypothesis is still valid.

One of the difficulties in all learning experiments is that the animals do not learn precisely what the experimenter wishes them to learn. The sensory input associated with being placed in the test apparatus may also be incorporated into the animal's memory, and salient features of that experience may become recognizable (learned). That is, the animal may respond to a novel environment in the same sense that it does to a structured learning task. There has been a report of just such a circum-stance. Thirsty rats were injected with radioactive uridine and then placed in a test cage in which water was delivered by a loud mechanical activation of a valve. Three control groups were also studied. The first was placed in the same test cage but received no water when the valve was activated. The second was left in its home cage to drink water at will, and the third was left in the home cage without water. After 1 hour the brains were removed from all the rats and dissected to obtain specific regions, from which RNA was extracted. Compared to the third control group (those in the home cage without water) all other rats had an increased incorporation of label into RNA extracted from the hippocampus, but not from other brain regions. Moreover, these results were obtainable only with rats newly arrived from the supplier; those rats that were allowed to adapt to the home cage for a week or more showed no differences in labeled uridine incorporated into RNA, whether they were experimental or control animals. The researchers concluded that the novelty of the experience was associated with the increased incorporation into RNA where it occurred with the newly arrived rats. They pointed out that the hippocampus is known to have a theta rhythm of electrical activity (an EEG frequency slower than the predominant pattern), which has been found to arise in early learning experiences or in novel experiences. They therefore speculated that the increased label incorporation into RNA might be correlated with the theta rhythm.

These and other experiments demonstrate that the normal learning process is associated in some way with increased incorporation of radioactive precursors into RNA under such test conditions, and presumably therefore with increased metabolic activity of RNA under normally occurring conditions. However, it has been reported by many investigators that inhibitors of RNA or protein synthesis prevent storage in long-term memory but do not interfere with learning. There is an implied inconsistency, for it seems unlikely that changes in RNA metabolism would normally accompany the insight phase and yet not be required for learning. It could be, of course, that the increased RNA metabolism subserves a restorative function which is ultimately required, but it is not obligatory, during the brief time insight is developing. Another possibility is that the increased RNA metabolism results from the completion of the insight process and is required only for the formation of long-term memory. Figure 10-1 illustrates a sequential model of memory formation. Short-term storage leads to intermediate-term storage which in turn leads to long-term storage. If the above speculation about the function of increased RNA metabolism is correct, the model of Figure 10-2 may be more appropriate.

It is a parallel model, in that the process of long-term storage is postulated to begin immediately with the learning experience and to require increased RNA metabolism in its initial stages. Short-term memory would of course also occur early in the learning experience, but it would only be convertible to intermediate-term memory. If these speculations are correct the neurochemical correlates of short- and intermediate-term memory would not include changes in RNA metabolism.

It is clear that, although this field of study is still largely undeveloped, further progress is to be anticipated from the shared efforts of researchers in the several brain sciences. The situation is not unlike that of the studies of chemical imprinting (Chapter 6); many leads are now under active exploration and there is a sense of progress and promise, but the clarifying experiments are still to come.

State-Dependent Learning

Learning in experimental animals occurs under a variety of conditions which are partially under the control of the experimenters. The strength or duration of an aversive stimulus may be varied, or the drive to obtain food or water may be increased by prior deprivation. When an inhibitor of cerebral neurochemical processes is injected, a great deal of attention is devoted to avoiding a level of general toxicity that may be sufficiently great so as to impair all performance. It would seem that what one ought to try most carefully to avoid is to attempt to measure learning during a generalized drug state. Surprisingly, just such efforts have led to a new way to study learning. Although the theoretical foundations are not yet understood, the existence of the observed phenomena has extensive applications to many human activities.

When an experimental animal learns while under the influence of a drug, its subsequent performance in the drug-free state is considerably worse than either its own performance just after finishing the learning trial or the performance of a control animal that has had the same learning without exposure to the drug. This by itself would hardly seem surprising. However, if the animal which has learned the task while under the influence of the drug is retested, not in the drug-free state but after a second injection of the same drug, its performance is as good as the control. In general it is found that if the state of the animal (either drug or no drug) is the same during learning and retesting, performance is better than if a change in state (from drug to no drug, or the reverse) has occurred.

These unexpected results were first observed 35 years ago and have since been extensively documented and expanded. Closely related is the phenomenon known as drug discrimination. The simplest example is that of a rat taught to choose the left branch of a Y-maze while in the drug-free state and the right branch, in response to the same cue, while in the drug state. The coexistence of the two responses, coupled with the observations that the process of learning the second response was neither retarded nor enhanced as a result of having learned the first response, led to the term "dissociated learning."

Several hypotheses have been advanced to explain these phenomena. The earliest suggested that drug-free and drug-accompanied learning occur in different brain regions. Subsequently other researchers suggested that the drug state favored some neural pathways at particular synaptic junctions. Others proposed that the drug state impaired cognition so that the animal perceived only some of the stimuli associated with the task and therefore learned a simpler task than the drug-free control. According to other researchers the drug acted as a conditioned stimulus by producing physiological changes which were perceived as internal cues.

At the present time, during which none of these hypotheses is predominant, intensive experimental efforts are underway to define the phenomena more precisely. A careful review of many studies has shown that only those drugs that penetrate the blood-brain barrier and act on the CNS will lead to a discriminative response; peripheral effects of these drugs apparently do not contribute to dissociated learning.

The phenomenom of dissociated learning has been

employed to categorize various drugs. Thus, an animal trained to seek food in the left arm of a Y-maze after receiving pento-barbital, and in the right arm of the maze after receiving saline, could then be tested with other drugs to determine which elicited the left-turn behavior and which others led to the right-turn response. By this technique it was found that, in addition to other barbituates, chloral hydrate, meprobamate, and chlordiaze-poxide all produced the pentobarbital response, while chlor-promazine, amphetamine, nicotine, and tetrahydrocannabinol (the active ingredient in marijuana) produced the saline response. This does not mean that the latter group of drugs is as innocuous as saline but rather that their discriminative properties were unlike those of the barbituates in this particular experiment.

In other studies it was demonstrated that dissociated learning could be produced by each of the drugs that gave the saline response in the experiment just described. For example, when administration of nicotine led to dissociation with respect to saline controls, the large group of drugs that produced the saline response included pentobarbital, caffeine, amphetamine, and adrenaline. It is important at this point to recall the design of the experiment, since the reference to pentobarbital both as a drug which produces dissociated learning and as a drug which is not different from saline would seem at first to be inconsistent.

Table 10-1 summarizes the design. Procedures 1, 4, and 5

Table 10-1
STATE-DEPENDENT LEARNING

Procedure	Drug Utilized in Learning	Drug Utilized in Retesting	Result
1	Pentobarbital	Pentobarbital	+
2	Pentobarbital	Saline or nicotine	−
3	Saline or nicotine	Pentobarbital	−
4	Saline	Saline	+
5	Nicotine	Nicotine	+
6	Nicotine	Saline	−
7	Saline	Nicotine	−

Good learning is signified by "+," deficient learning by "−."

require learning and retesting in the same state; in all others there is a different drug state going from learning to testing. Nicotine is not a satisfactory replacement for pentobarbital (line 2), nor is pentobarbital an adequate replacement for nicotine (line 6) when going from learning to retesting. The same kind of statement is true for many pairs of drugs, from which it may be concluded that the mechanisms of dissociation by any particular drug must involve specific neural pathways and that drug alterations of any one of several such pathways lead to dissociation. This strongly implies that learning and storage occur through the mediation of alternative neuronal circuits and should not be ascribed to any one morphological location or functional pathway.

Similar phenomena are demonstrable in humans with several drugs. The tests, as with experimental animals, require demonstration of a memory for learned tasks. It is usual to require that the subject learn unrelated word groups, or related pairs of words, and then test for remembrance up to a day later. By such techniques it has been shown that some of the barbituates produce state-dependent learning. Of particular interest, however, are studies with alcohol. A number of investigations have demonstrated that some degree of state-dependent learning is produced by alcohol although alcoholics and nonalcoholics do not appear to differ in these tests. The interest in alcohol stems from the well-known occurrence of alcoholic blackouts, in which a sizable amnesia for events occurring during alcohol intake are reported in the subsequent drug-free state. At the present time there is no good evidence that these blackouts are a variation of state-dependent learning. However, the question is still under experimental investigation.

Although there have been few experimental studies of state-dependent learning in humans, it has been the subject of much speculative attention. For example, some have wondered whether the widespread use of amphetamines during intensive preparation for examinations may lead to a state-dependent effect in which subsequent recall during the examination is worse than it would have been without the drug. Since drug use, whether legally sanctioned or otherwise, is widespread among humans, many potential state-dependent effects may be anticipated. Further research is needed to explore such possibilities.

PART THREE

*Chemistry and Uncontrolled
Behavior*

11

Transient Behavioral Changes Produced by Ingested Substances

IT BEGAN SUDDENLY one afternoon with a peculiar sensation of restlessness and dizziness. Soon the shapes of people and things around him appeared to change. Unable to concentrate, and in a dreamlike state, he went home, driven by an irresistible urge to lie down and sleep. Ordinary daylight became unpleasantly intense. Lying down with his eyes closed, fantastic intensely colored images of extraordinary plasticity seemed to surge toward him. The experience lasted 2 hours, after which he recovered completely.

Such is the account of the first recorded LSD trip, as experienced by its discoverer, Dr. Albert Hofman. He had been synthesizing related compounds and had accidentally absorbed a very small amount of the substance. The effects he described were soon confirmed and extended with controlled studies, and it became apparent that a drug-induced psychosis could be produced by microgram quantities of LSD. Further studies with other substances led to the terms "hallucinogenic" and "psychotomimetic" to describe the behavioral and psychological states resulting from their ingestion.

153

There are, however, reproducible differences in the effects produced by different members of this group of substances. Although the drugs are administered orally and thus available to the entire body, the site of the effect is almost certainly the CNS. The variety of human behavior produced by these substances is reminiscent of the various effects in experimental animals produced by the direct intracerebral injection of other drugs. The same general conclusions hold; the specificity of behavioral effects of the various psychotomimetics strongly implies a specific chemical organization of the human brain. The details of the neurochemical-behavioral correlates constitute the subject matter of this chapter.

Amphetamines

It has long been the hope of researchers investigating the possible causes and treatments of psychotic states that a "model psychosis" would be recognized. By this is meant a brief drug-induced psychotic state whose symptoms are largely indistinguishable from those that characterize one of the major psychotic illnesses. The advantages of the identification of a drug-induced behavior as a model psychosis are readily apparent: if the two states are virtually the same and the immediate cause of one is known (specific drug intake), then its neurophysiological and neurochemical consequences can be studied extensively in animals with a view toward identifying those changes that are necessarily correlated with the observed behavior. Once such correlations are established it may then be possible to devise an appropriate chemical intervention that would be an effective treatment for the human disease state.

It is a widely reported observation that patients hospitalized for amphetamine overdose often have psychotic symptoms which are difficult to distinguish from those of acute paranoid schizophenia. Symptoms common to the two states are reported to include paranoid ideation, ideas of reference (the notion that entirely independent activities, such as television programs, are really directed at the subject), distortions of body image, and less frequently with the amphetamine-induced psychosis—auditory and visual hallucinations and some disorganization of thought processes. Because of the close similarity in symptomatology amphetamine has been studied extensively in patients, in volunteer human subjects, and in several animal species.

Psychotic symptoms result from chronic use of relatively high doses of amphetamine. Other behavioral changes are seen with much smaller doses. Anorexia is produced at all dose levels. The moderate use of amphetamine in weight loss programs is, of course, well documented. The anorexia is more severe with higher doses and is followed by a ravenous appetite on withdrawal of the drug. This appetite rebound should be contrasted with the results of nondrug induced starvation, in which appetite is usually reduced as weight loss proceeds. Insomnia, another well-known and prominent effect of amphetamine ingestion, is also dependent upon dose levels. Subjects who have self-administered large doses of amphetamine intraveneously have been reported to go without sleep for 6 days. The REM phase of sleep is reduced, and there is a compensating REM rebound upon withdrawal. In addition to appetite and sleep rebound, withdrawal is accompanied by more serious effects. Lowered mood states, sometimes of the intensity of severe depressions, with sudden unpredictable suicide attempts, have been reported.

Amphetamine intake in humans is sometimes accompanied by pronounced changes in sexuality, usually in the direction of increased sexual drive. Unprovoked violence, sometimes having a psychotic quality, may also occur with heavy use.

The behavioral activation resulting from amphetamine administration to animals is considered to be analogous to the human effects listed above. In addition stereotypic behavior, such as repetitive and apparently purposeless sniffing, licking, and biting, results from amphetamine administration to animals. Stereotypy has also been reported in humans; it is manifested in acts such as repetitive polishing of an automobile for hour after hour, meticulous sorting of small objects with no apparent purpose, and continuous doodling for hours. Thus, with the range of human behavioral changes produced by amphetamines and with apparently similar effects in animals, the "model psychosis" aspect of amphetamine use has led to a great deal of experimental investigation.

Initially it was thought that amphetamines merely released or augmented psychoses in schizophrenic subjects. However, several studies have now shown that normal volunteers, screened to exclude any subjects with schizophrenic symptoms, will become psychotic within 1 day if given repeated doses of amphetamine totaling several hundred milligrams. The symptoms of the induced psychoses were very similar to those of patients undergoing an acute paranoid schizophrenic episode. The psychoses cleared completely within 3 days under these controlled laboratory conditions. The same studies also rule out starvation and sleep deprivation as contributing causes, since the induced psychoses were observable within 1 day.

Further understanding required detailed animal experimentation with each of the stereoisomers of amphetamine (see Figure 11-1). Since one of the carbon atoms in the side chain

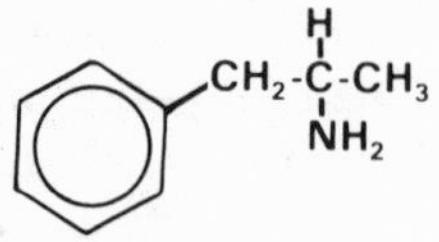

d-amphetamine

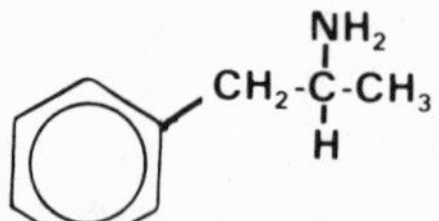

l-amphetamine

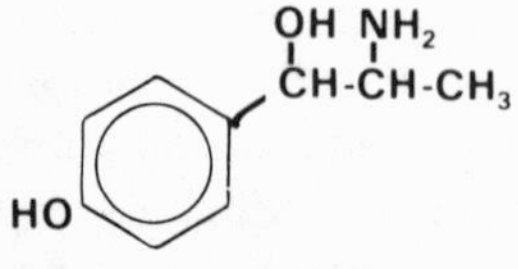

Para hydroxy norephedrine

Figure 11-1. Amphetamine stereoisomers and an amphetamine derivative. Benzedrine is *dl*-amphetamine.

bonds to four different chemical groups (the amino group, the hydrogen atom, the methyl group, and the benzyl group) there are two geometric arrangements that are possible. One of these, d-amphetamine is also known as Dexedrine. The mixture *dl-* amphetamine, is Benzedrine. As is usual with stereoisomeric substances, the mixture of the *d* and *l* forms is most readily available and thus has been employed most frequently. However, the separate isomers have also been studied behaviorally and neurochemically with some interesting results.

A large body of evidence indicates that norepinephrine is involved in the CNS actions of amphetamine. Initially it was postulated that amphetamine released norepinephrine from storage sites in the nerve terminals and that amphetamine effects were therefore to be regarded as augmented norepinephrine effects. More recently this view has been subject to refinement and revision.

Reserpine is a drug which depletes the CNS of norepinephrine by causing release, and subsequent nonfunctional metabolism, from the storage sites (see Chapters 8 and 10). When reserpine is given to animals prior to amphetamine administration, psychomotor stimulation is maintained and sometimes even augmented, over the level of activity resulting from amphetamine alone. This observation suggested that, if amphetamine action did depend upon norepinephrine, the ongoing synthesis of norepinephrine, rather than the stored reserve, might be the relevant factor.

The enzyme inhibitor, alpha methyl tyrosine, is known to interfere with the synthesis of norepinephrine by blocking the enzyme tyrosine hydroxylase, which converts tyrosine to norepinephrine (see Chapter 8). When alpha methyl tyrosine is administered prior to amphetamine, no psychomotor stimulation results. Thus ongoing synthesis of norepinephrine does seem to be required for amphetamine action. However, since dopamine is a precursor of norepinephrine and is also depleted by alpha methyl tyrosine, it was necessary to distinguish between these substances as mediators of the amphetamine effect. This was accomplished in rats by surgically destroying a region of the substantia nigra which accounts for many of the dopamine-containing neurons. When this was done it was found that amphetamine administration still caused psychomotor activation but that stereotyped behavior was no longer elicited. Thus amphetamine acts on at least two neural systems: the nigro-striatal system, producing stereotypy, and the norepinephrine projection pathways, leading to psychomotor activation.

The norepinephrine effects were investigated in more detail by employing the technique of self-stimulation. By this technique electrodes, chronically implanted at various regions in a rat brain, deliver a small stimulation current when the rat presses a lever. When the electrode is in the median forebrain bundle (a group of fibers, some containing norepinephrine, going between limbic system structures, the hypothalamus, and the midbrain tegmentum), the resulting stimulus is apparently pleasurable to the rats, for they will engage in repetitive lever pressing to obtain stimulation. The frequency of self-stimulation is increased by substances known to cause rapid release of synaptic norepinephrine, and by d-amphetamine as well. Dopamine beta hydroxylase, the enzyme that converts dopamine to norepinephrine (Chapter 8), is blocked by the drug disulfiram and by diethyldithiocarbamate (DEDTC), a metabolite of disulfiram. This substance also suppresses self-stimulation, as would be expected if self-stimulation requires norepinephrine. The subsequent injection of norepinephrine into the lateral ventricles will partially restore self-stimulation toward the normal base-line level. Dopamine and serotonin are without effect in this regard. If DEDTC is administered prior to amphetamine, self-stimulation is blocked. Addition of norepinephrine along with amphetamine, subsequent to DEDTC injection, will produce the augmented level of self-stimulation characteristic of amphetamine alone. These results clearly demonstrate that newly supplied norepinephrine is required for self-stimulation and that amphetamine augments its activity. Normally the requirement is met by new synthesis of norepinephrine; in these experiments it can also be met by adding norepinephrine to the lateral ventricles, from which it travels to the depleted neurons. The researchers assume that the new norepinephrine is stored in a labile functional pool from which it is readily displaced by amphetamine.

The same researchers were able to show that norepinephrine was released from neurons in the amygdala by a high rate of self-stimulation, and also by amphetamine. They speculated that norepinephrine, released from the amygdala in response to amphetamine, may have a disinhibiting effect on neuronal activity. This suggestion was based on experiments in which rats were simultaneously rewarded with milk and punished with foot shock for lever-pressing behavior. Under such conditions the animals suppressed some lever pressing, tolerating just enough foot shock to obtain the amount of milk desired. When the amygdala was subsequently damaged slightly by insertion of a cannula, the suppressed behavior was partially released and lever pressing increased. Direct application of a crystal of norepinephrine to the amygdala through the cannula caused a further release of the suppressed behavior, from which they suggested that norepinephrine, released from storage by amphetamine, may release other modes of suppressed behavior, thereby producing the observed behavioral activation.

The molecular mechanism by which amphetamine displaces norepinephrine is not known. However, it is known that para hydroxy norephedrine (see Figure 11-1), a metabolite of amphetamine, is a false transmitter in the peripheral nervous system. It may also have such a role in the CNS.

D-amphetamine has been shown to inhibit the entry of norepinephrine into synaptosomes, the enclosed portion of nerve endings that are formed in the process of homogenizing nerve-tissue (see Chapter 8). In this respect it is about 10 times as effective as the *l* isomer. Thus enhanced release of newly formed norepinephrine, inhibitions of re-uptake of norepinephrine, and false transmitter activity must be considered among the mechanisms by which amphetamine produces its effects. Since the effects are varied, ranging from insomnia and anorexia through psychomotor activation and stereotypy to psychosis, there is room for more than one mechanism.

The effects requiring interference with norepinephrine appear to be specific to the *d* isomer, which is 10 times more potent than the *l* form in producing psychomotor activation in rats. In contrast stereotypic behavior, involving dopamine, is produced by either d- or l-amphetamine. It was therefore important to determine whether one isomer was a more potent human psychomimetic agent than the other. It has been reported that they are approximately equally potent in producing psychoses of similar qualitative nature, suggesting that dopamine systems are involved in the psychotic behavior. These observations have been used to support a dopamine hypothesis of schizophrenia (see Chapter 13).

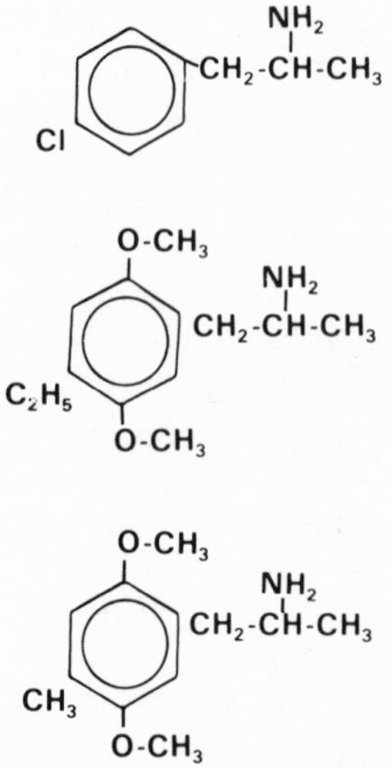

Para chloroamphetamine

Dimethoxy ethyl amphetamine (DOET)

Dimethoxy methyl amphetamine (DOM)

Figure 11-2. Some amphetamine derivatives.

Many amphetamine derivatives have been synthesized and studied for specific behavioral effects (see Figure 11-2). Para chloroamphetamine produces insomnia and has a more potent anorexigenic effect than amphetamine but it has no apparent effect on norepinephrine or dopamine. It does lower the concentration of serotonin and its metabolites in rat and guinea pig brains. Since serotonin has been linked to sleep mechanisms, the insomnia produced by para chloroamphetamine may relate to its actions on serotonin function. By implication the anorexigenic effects of amphetamine, as well as the insomnia-producing activity, may similarly be due to interaction with serotonin. If so, this substance acts on three important biogenic amines (serotonin, norepinephrine, and dopamine), and psychoses resulting from high-dose levels may be the product of all of these interactions.

Two other derivatives, DOET and DOM (also known as

STP), have been studied in volunteer subjects at low doses (see Figure 11-2). Subjective effects produced by DOET were compared with those produced by amphetamine. Both substances were reported to produce euphoria, but at the low-dose level which was used subjects reported feelings of insight, greater awareness of body image, difficulty in concentrating, and impatience with psychological tests when receiving DOET, but not when receiving amphetamine. In contrast, the same subjects reported that their concentration was better than normal when receiving amphetamine, but not with DOET. All tests were done "double blind," without either the subject or the observer knowing which drug was administered. When different doses of DOET were compared, it was found that, at doses five times the minimum needed to produce any subjective effects, no hallucinatory activity was reported. In contrast, DOM was psychotomimetic at comparable doses.

LSD

Many clinical studies, both with normal volunteers and with patients in various therapeutic settings, have essentially confirmed the elements of the LSD experience as first recorded by Dr. Hofman. These range from somatic effects such as dizziness and nausea, through a variety of distortions of sensory and proprioceptive input, to more complex effects on mood and thought processes. What appears characteristic among the extensive reports available is the apparent episodic nature of all of the changes.

Thus, the simplest visual effect is blurred vision, but the blurring clears and reappears randomly throughout the experience. The visual field is often described as being filled with strange objects, and three-dimensional space appears alternately to contract and enlarge. Walls appear as undulating objects, sometimes moving in on the subject. Angles are distorted and changes in space perception occur. Light appears to fluctuate in intensity. Similar auditory effects occur, but to a lesser degree. There is an altered sensitivity to sound, which seems to pulsate, making localization of voices difficult. The separation between sensory modalities sometimes disappears—subjects will report that they "saw" rippling waves when a telephone rang.

Tactile perceptions are also subject to fluctuation. Textures may be described as very coarse or very fine, or as unreal. Temperature sensitivity is altered, the normal environment may be perceived as too hot or too cold. Changes in perception of pressure and weight occur—an arm felt so light that it "floated" upwards. The body image is altered—a subject will report that he "saw" his body on the chair while he floated out of it. This too is a fluctuating feeling.

Time sometimes appears speeded up, sometimes slowed down. It may also appear to run backwards, as if the subject were viewing a film that ran backwards. Thus he may first be aware that he is drinking from a glass, and then he becomes aware that he has picked it up.

Thought processes are altered. There is a shorter concentration span, unrelated thoughts are interposed in a conversation, the mind appears to wander, thoughts are uncontrolled, and memory defects appear. There are ideas of reference, delusions, and bizarre ideas. Mood changes include euphoria or a flat affect. There may be increased fear or a sense of a transcendental experience.

There is apparently selective recall of some aspects of the LSD experience. During the period of drug activity the subject may report that he feels less friendly, more aggressive or agitated, or depressed. Much later, he will recall the experience as illuminating and pleasurable. He will rarely recall psychotic symptoms.

Overall, it appears that the LSD experience is characterized at least in part by a scrambling of the normal information-processing aspects of the CNS. Sensory modalities intrude upon each other's domain; the temporal sequence of events can be lost, suggesting a disorganization of short-term memory; sensory information is alternately overweighted and underweighted (undulating walls, variable intensities of sound and light); and thoughts are verbalized without reference to preceding or succeeding thoughts. As several investigators have pointed out, the experience can be psychotomimetic or psychedelic, depending upon the subject's environment. Considering the profound disruption of CNS processes that occurs, it is unlikely that anyone subjected to such challenges will be able to view the experience in an undramatic way.

From the neurochemical point of view, the extensive disorganization of so many aspects of CNS information processing suggests that either LSD has targeted on some neural pathways or regions responsible for overall control of impulse sequencing or that its effects are disseminated widely over many neurons.

Before reviewing the various molecular and neurophysiological hypotheses of LSD activity, it is useful to focus on one of the most intriguing aspects of this substance—the extraordinary low concentration at which it is effective. It has been found that injection of a dose as low as 25 micrograms in a normal human will produce a clear behavioral response. The quantity subsequently available to the brain is reduced by rapid metabolic conversion to inactive products. For example, in rats 60% to 80% of an injected dose was metabolized by the liver and excreted in the bile within 3 hours, at which time the concentration of LSD in the brain was less than half of that found in the blood plasma. Only 1/10,000 of the injected dose was found in the brain, which had the lowest concentration of any tissue studied. The concentration in the blood in humans is reduced by half every 3 hours, and amounts to 6 to 7 micrograms per liter of plasma 1/2 hour after injection of 150 micrograms. If the distribution between the blood and brain that occurs for the rat is also true for humans, it can be estimated that less than 2% of the dose is present in the human brain 3 hours after intravenous injection. Thus, if a 25-microgram dose is given, it can be estimated that the number of molecules of LSD present in the brain 3 hours later is 10^{15}. If they were equally distributed at each of the 10^{13} synaptic junctions, and nowhere else, there would only be 100 molecules per synapse. The true average number per synapse is likely to be much less since LSD is found in the cytoplasm as well, and it probably also enters the glial cells. Thus it is likely that any hypothesis postulating that the synapses are the sites of action of LSD would be encumbered by the requirement to attribute such a potent effect to less than 10 molecules at each synapse. It is known that there are differences in regional concentration within the brain; the hippocampus has the highest and cerebellum the lowest concentration of the several regions studied. But even so the average synaptic content is only going to be raised by 10 to 20 molecules.

The probability, then, is that there are a few specific target cells, in effect LSD receptors, which accumulate a sufficient number of molecules to significantly perturb some local neurochemical processes. Such neurons would then have some vital role in the sense that they would organize the flow of information between many other neurons. With this background it is intriguing to consider some results of a recent neurophysiological study. The researchers determined the spontaneous rate of firing of neuronal units in the rat midbrain raphe nuclei. They then observed that after injection of LSD the spontaneous activity of all of these cells came to a halt and then gradually recovered. Since nearby cells in the reticular formation and pontine nuclei were not affected, it was concluded that the LSD effect was specific for the raphe nuclei, which produce most of the brain serotonin. LSD was known to reduce the utilization of serotonin, as evidenced by an increase in its concentration and a concomitant fall in the concentration of 5-hydroxyindole acetic acid, a metabolite.

It was also observed that, just as the LSD effect was specific for the anatomical site, so also did that site respond specifically to LSD and not at all to other substances such as amphetamine, chlorpromazine, norepinephrine, or serotonin. Other substances were found that were inhibitory, although less potent. They include an LSD derivative, 2-brom LSD, dimethyltryptamine (DMT), and mescaline (see Figure 11-3). However, in contrast to LSD, which inhibited all neurons in the raphe nuclei, the other substances were specific for some, but not all, of the raphe neurons.

This does not mean that the site of action of LSD has been found. It is possible that further studies will reveal regions where LSD increases ongoing activity, or alters the threshold to specific transmitters. However, it is a significant beginning in a long search whose conclusion may signal a substantial advance in our concepts about neural information processing.

Anticholinergics

The symptom complex is frequently described as a "toxic delirium." CNS symptoms include incoherence and confusion, auditory and visual hallucinations, apprehension and paranoid ideation, and not infrequently a retrograde amnesia for the

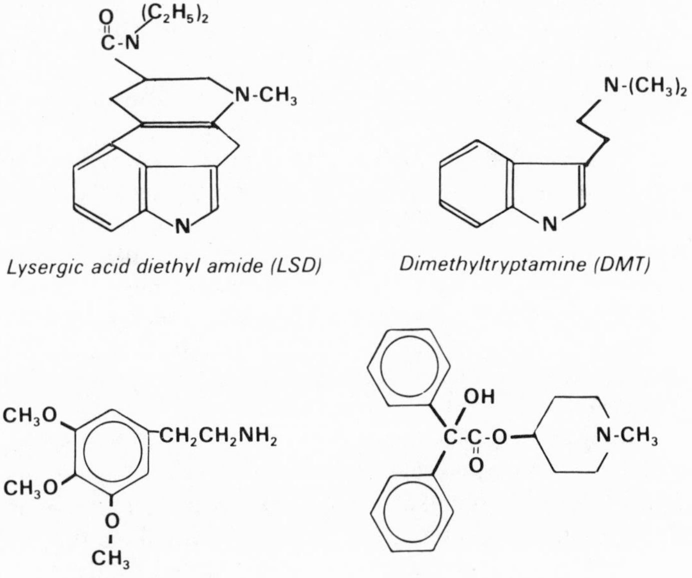

Lysergic acid diethyl amide (LSD) · *Dimethyltryptamine (DMT)* · *Mescaline* · *Methyl piperidyl benzilate*

Figure 11-3. Structures of some psychotomimetic substances.

episode. Assaultive behavior may also occur. The visual hallucinations are described as vivid, involving people, animals, and crawling objects. In the latter case there is a similarity to the delirium tremens state that results from alcohol intoxication. Picking and grasping motions are associated with the hallucinations. At least to the extent that the hallucinations involve integrated images these psychotomimetic experiences are different from those produced by LSD. Other differences include the generally frightening nature of the anticholinergic-induced mental state, the lack of any overlap of response to visual and auditory input, and the relatively frequent occurrence of auditory hallucinations involving distinct voices and musical instruments.

Anticholinergic drugs, which occur in some solanaceous plants, have been employed for more than 2,000 years to evoke prophesies, materialize demons, attain visions, reduce pain, and poison enemies. Atropa belladonna (deadly nightshade), Hyoscyamus niger (black henbane), and Datura stramonium (Jimsonweed, thorn apple) contain atropine and scopolamine, substances which in appropriate conditions and small doses have had extensive medical usage.

Acetylcholine serves as a transmitter for CNS neurons and for peripheral neurons as well. It is the transmitter for that part of the autonomic nervous system known as the parasympathetic system. This system is composed of some cranial and sacral nerves, the ganglia at which they synapse, and their postganglionic fibers. Thus acetylcholine is the preganglionic transmitter and also the transmitter at the junction between the postganglionic fiber and the cell which it innervates. Acetylcholine also serves as the preganglionic transmitter for the sympathetic nervous system, for which adrenaline is the postganglionic transmitter.

Among the several kinds of target cells of the parasympathetic system, muscle cells are differentiated according to whether they are striated skeletal muscle cells or smooth muscle cells. (Smooth, or involuntary, muscle, is found along the length of the gastrointestinal tract, and it is innervated by the sympathetic as well as by the parasympathetic system.) Release of acetylcholine at the neuromuscular junction, whether of striated or smooth muscle, results in contraction. The acetylcholine-stimulated contraction of smooth muscle is blocked by atropine, but not curare, while skeletal muscle contraction is blocked by curare, but not atropine. Two kinds of receptors for acetylcholine are therefore indicated. Muscarine can substitute for the action of acetylcholine in stimulating smooth muscle contraction; hence this type of receptor is termed "muscarinic." Nicotine can substitute for acetylcholine in skeletal muscle contraction; hence the second receptor is termed "nicotinic."

In addition to smooth muscle, muscarinic acetylcholine receptors exist at glands such as the salivary and lacrimal glands. Release of acetylcholine at the neuroreceptor junction causes increased secretion. In general, actions driven in one direction by parasympathetic fibers are counterbalanced by sympathetic fibers. For example, the pupil of the eye contracts (meiosis) or expands (midriasis) in response to parasympathetic or sympathetic input. These relationships lead to a number of predictable consequences when atropine, scopolamine, or other anticholinergics specific for muscarinic receptors act on peripheral tissue. Midriasis, lack of salivation, a flushed dry skin, and increased heart rate are among the prominent peripheral effects of the anti-cholinergics. Since many anticholinergics pass through the blood-brain barrier slowly, peripheral effects usually predominate unless the dose taken is 5 to 10 times the amount required for valid medical purposes. However, there are some CNS effects caused by scopolamine at low-dose levels, as indicated by its use as a sleep-inducing medication. At the higher dose levels the extensive symptoms of toxic delirium are easily produced.

There are some synthetic anticholinergics that readily pass the blood-brain barrier. These substances, known as piperidyl benzilate esters (Figure 11-3), have very potent CNS effects. Severe disruption of thought processes occur, along with disorganization and disorientation. Even after substantial recovery, some confusion may persist for days. The experiences are generally regarded as frightening and not psychedelic.

The neurochemical mechanism is presumed to involve competition between acetylcholine and an anticholinergic at a postsynaptic muscarinic receptor. This postulate is supported by the effective use of a cholinesterase inhibitor, physostigmine, to treat the toxicity resulting from an overdose of anticholinergics. Since the enzyme inhibitor limits the synaptic metabolism of acetylcholine, the large increase in the concentration of acetyl-choline that occurs allows more effective competition with the anticholinergic substance for binding at the receptor site, thus restoring the synapse to its normal function. Studies of subcellular distribution are consistent with this view in that they show a close association in localization of acetylcholine and the anticholi-nergics. Furthermore, it has been shown that direct application of acetylcholine to a microscopically small region of an animal brain, by a technique known as iontophoresis, has the same neurophysiological consequences as are obtained by stimulation of cholinergic pathways and that prior application of atropine and related substances blocks the effects of iontophoretically applied acetylcholine.

Opiates and Endorphins

The opium poppy, containing the alkaloid morphine, has

long been utilized as an analgesic drug in medical practice, and also as a source of euphoric experience. Much has been written about the addiction that accompanies prolonged morphine intake, and about the difficulty of withdrawal; these topics will not be elaborated upon here. However, the remarkable pain relieving properties of morphine and its diacetyl derivative, heroin, and other related alkaloids as well, have led many investigators to suspect that elucidation of the underlying neurochemical events would provide further important insights into brain organization. Pursuit of that goal has led to a rapid and largely unanticipated enlargment in our knowledge of brain chemistry.

There are a number of synthetic analogues of morphine based on minor modifications of the common chemical structure. Some of these have enhanced analgesic potency; others are antagonists to the action of morphine. All show stereospecificity. That is, one of a pair of isomers differing in spatial configuration about a single carbon atom will be active while the other member of the pair will show little or no activity. These facts—common chemical structure, sterospecificity, existence of specific antagonists, as well as the low doses required to produce pharmacological action—have led to the supposition that the brain contains specific receptors for the morphine alkaloids.

Within the past few years it has become possible to demonstrate the existence of such opiate receptors, and to describe their anatomical distribution within the human brain. It was found that structures comprising parts of the limbic system had the highest concentration, while regions such as the cerebellum had almost none at all. With this knowledge firmly secured, attention then turned to the likely possibility that the existence of such receptors implied the existence within the brain of normally occurring substances which would require such receptors. That is, it was suggested that the brain ought to contain naturally occurring opiates. The chemical structure of these postulated substances could not be inferred from the structure of morphine, but had to be determined independently.

The search for extracts of brain tissue that would have opiate-like activity proceeded methodically. Since opiates were known to reduce the contractions of smooth muscle tissue that can be produced by electrical stimulation, this property was utilized to screen each brain extract for such capacity. When such an extract was defined and was subjected to extensive purification and concentration, it was found to contain two peptides, each containing a sequence of five amino acids. These peptides were termed 'enkephalins'. One of them had as its constituent amino acids the sequence: tyrosine-glycine-glycine-phenylalanine-methionine. The second differed in that the amino acid leucine replaced methionine. The first substance was named 'methionine enkephalin' and the second one, 'leucine enkephalin'. Since such substances are easily synthesized by organic chemists, a number of variations were prepared so that there could be a comparison of relative analgesic potency. Tests in experimental animals showed that potency increased when the first glycine following tyrosine in the sequence was replaced by *d*-alanine, since this sequence was impervious to the action of normally occurring enzymes which degrade the peptides to inactive products.

The amino acid sequence of methionine enkephalin was noted by the research group that identified it to be identical to an amino acid sequence occurring within beta-lipotropin, a 91 amino acid peptide whose sequence had been determined 10 years earlier at another research center. Specifically, the sequence of amino acids which characterizes methionine enkephalin also occurs at amino acid positions 61 to 65 in the larger peptide, which had been found in the pituitary. It was soon discovered that extracts of the pituitary contain peptides, called endorphins, which have opiate potency. The peptide with the greatest opiate potency, known as beta-endorphin, has an amino acid sequence identical to that found in positions 61 to 91 of beta-lipotropin. Tests with experimental animals showed that the analgesic effects of successive doses of enkephalins or endorphins diminished unless the dose was increased. This phenomenon, known as tolerance, as well as the observation that physical dependence results from repeated doses, is characteristic of the effects of addictive drugs.

At doses less than one-hundredth of that required to produce analgesia in rats, beta-endorphin has been found to produce a muscular rigidity which resembled a catatonic state, and which could be counteracted by naloxone, a morphine antagonist. Beta-endorphin also produced hypothermia, while gamma-endorphin, a peptide whose amino acid sequence is identical with positions 61 to 77 of beta-lipotropin, produced hyperthermia. Enkephalins have been found to alter the firing rate of single neurons in rat brains and endorphins are believed to interact with cholinergic systems. From these and other observations the consensus is emerging that these peptides function as neurotransmitters.

The demonstration of the existence of endorphins and their specific receptors has stimulated the search for a neurophysiological role for other brain peptides. Behavioral effects have already been found for some of these. For example, thyrotropin-releasing hormone which can alter the fighting behavior of mice, is an effective agent in state-dependent learning, and decreases the length of time mice sleep after a standard dose of pentobarbital. Neurotensin, another peptide with a regional brain distribution similar to, but not identical with, that of endorphins, extends the pentobarbital sleeping time and inhibits the firing rate of neurons in the locus caeruleus. Although the exploration of this field has only recently begun, it is already clear that many different peptides have activity at the synaptic level. The possibility exists that at least some of them will be identified with specific behavioral effects.

Having demonstrated that there are receptors for the analgesic action of opiates, and that there are normally occurring peptides which have an analgesic affect, it now becomes reasonable to suppose that there are specific receptors for the euphoric action of opiates, and that normally occurring peptides having such euphoric affect will be identified. To carry the speculation one step further, if it becomes possible to demonstrate a variety of specific behavioral effects that can be attributed to individual peptides, perhaps some of the actions of the psychomimetic substances discussed earlier in this chapter will be found to provide useful clues to the specificity of behavioral control mechanisms normally available to the brain. And finally, can new peptides producing new forms of behavior be synthesized in the brain, perhaps in a feedback response to drugs that act on specific receptor sites? If so, long-term behavioral modification as a consequence of brief periods of drug ingestion can be anticipated.

There are many synthetic and naturally occurring substances whose ingestion leads to a variety of psychotomimetic experiences. The four groups discussed in this chapter were chosen to illustrate the range and specificity of behavioral effects, as well as the manifestly differing neurochemical sites of action. Since the desire for revelation and transcendental experience has existed throughout recorded history, it seems certain that continued self-experimentation will greet every new potential psychotomimetic drug. To the extent that this process leads to overdose requiring emergency medical or psychiatric care, we can be certain that a steady source of information about the drug's effects will be available to scientists as a result of the unfortunate experiences of the overdosed subjects. More important from the viewpoint of furthering our understanding of brain function are those safe and ethically acceptable controlled studies that yield valid scientific conclusions. The information obtained in this way points to details of brain organization that are unobtainable from any conceivable animal study. The results of the knowledge so obtained are important for the understanding and design of possible treatments for several categories of mental illness.

12

Affect and Endogenous Chemistry

THE CHEMICALLY INDUCED psychoses, as well as the psychotic episodes that accompany or characterize some mental illnesses, are states of CNS disorganization that are well beyond the usual range of occurrences attributable to normal fluctuations in neurochemical and neurophysiological control systems. In contrast, we all experience moments of anxiety, brief periods of agitation or lethargy, change of sleep patterns, occasional "low" feelings, or inexplicable elation. These and other descriptors of variations in normal affect appear in intensified and extended form in manic-depressive disease. It is widely assumed that there is a continuum of affect and that the same neurochemical and neurophysiological controls underlie the whole range of affective behavior.

The following chapter will deal in detail with the correlations between altered neurochemistry and some mental illnesses; at this time it will be useful to explore those neurochemical events that are presumed to relate causally to the affective state. Since it is endogenous chemistry, rather than the effects of exogenous substances, that is postulated to be causally related to affect, proof of the cause and effect relationship is exceedingly difficult to obtain. There are few acceptable experiments which will vary the brain content of the putative causal agent; although therapeutic drugs are presumed to do so, they may act at various sites, altering concentrations more at one site than at another, or they may have multiple neurochemical actions.

Even though the difficulties are formidable, a hypothesis has developed over the past 15 years that relates the range of affect, from deep depression through normal mood variations to overt mania, to the effective levels of some of the amine transmitters. Evidence for and against this hypothesis will be reviewed in the following chapter. A brief outline of the hypothesis, given below, is followed by a detailed examination of the interrelation between various control systems.

The essence of the hypothesis is that neural pathways which utilize the amines as synaptic transmitters are centrally involved in the affective state and that affect is depressed or raised according to whether the amines are in short supply or are present in excess. More specifically, it is postulated that only that portion of the biogenic amine store that is available for functional utilization at the synapse is related to the affective state.

Figure 12-1 represents the schematic conceptualization of the

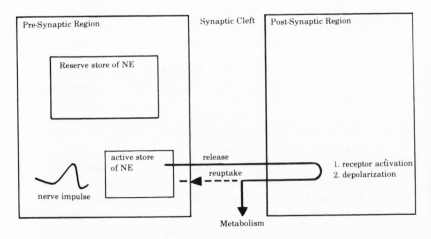

Figure 12-1. Schematic representation of events at a norepinephrine-containing nerve terminal.

hypothesis. A biogenic amine, for example norepinephrine, is largely stored at a reserve location in the nerve terminal; a much smaller portion is stored at some active site. When a propagated nerve impulse arrives at the terminal region a portion of the norepinephrine at the active site is released into the synapse, where it rapidly moves to the postsynaptic membrane, activates a receptor region, and returns by diffusion and re-uptake to the presynaptic terminal. The activated receptor initiates events that lead to depolarization of the postsynaptic membrane. After a number of such transmissions the postsynaptic neuron fires off a new nerve impulse (see Chapter 8). All factors that reduce the norepinephrine available to the synapse, as well as those that render the postsynpatic membrane insensitive, are postulated to result in a lower affective state. Control of the available transmitter can be effected at several points in the synthetic pathway, at the storage and release sites, by the enzymes that function in the synaptic cleft, and finally by the re-uptake mechanism.

Regulation of Biogenic Amines in the CNS

Regulation of the amine transmitter starts with the biosynthetic process. Figure 8-2 outlines the chemical events of dopamine and norepinephrine synthesis; an analogous sequence for serotonin synthesis is outlined in Figure 12-2. The first step in the intraneuronal synthesis of dopamine and norepinephrine is the substitution of a hydroxyl group for a hydrogen atom in the aromatic ring of the amino acid, L-tyrosine. The product is 3, 4 dihydroxyphenylalanine, otherwise known as L-DOPA. The conversion of tyrosine to L-DOPA is catalyzed by the enzyme tyrosine hydroxylase. Because this enzymatic step is rate limiting (it is the slowest pathway in the biosynthetic sequence), it has been studied intensively as an obvious control point in the synthesis of the two amine transmitters.

Tyrosine hydroxylase, which is found only in neural tissue, is located both in the perikaryon and in the nerve terminal. Its activity is subject to instantaneous regulation by feedback control and to long-term regulation by synthesis of new enzyme molecules. Various feedback control substances exist (see the discussion of feedback inhibition in Chapter 2). Some of these, such as norepinephirne and dopamine, produce their effect by competing with tetrahydropteridine, the cofactor required for enzy-

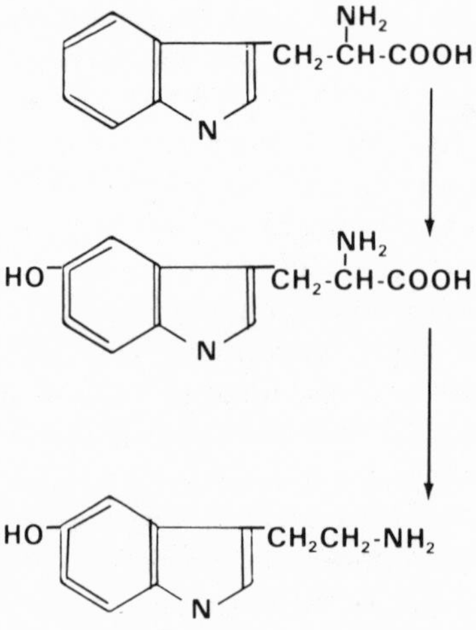

Tryptophan

5-hydroxy tryptophan

Serotonin

Figure 12-2. Synthesis of Serotonin from Tryptophan.

matic function. Others, which compete with tyrosine for binding by the enzyme, include alpha methyl tyrosine, phenylalanine, 3,5-diiodotyrosine (a metabolite of thyroxine), and other aromatic amino acids. To the extent that norepinephrine is synthesized in nerve terminals, feedback inhibition of significant proportions implies that a major part of the tyrosine hydroxylase is located in the terminals rather than in the perikaryon.

The amount of tyrosine hydroxylase found in neurons is ultimately related to its gene-directed synthesis. Reserpine, a drug that has been used extensively by pharmacologists to control hypertension, has been shown to produce an increase in the quantity of tyrosine hydroxylase found in the adrenals, the superior cervical ganglia, and the brainstem. The increase develops slowly and reaches a maximum in perikarya about 3 days after reserpine administration. Appearance of increased enzyme activity in nerve terminals occurs 2 days later. The drugs, actinomycin, which blocks the DNA-directed synthesis of RNA, and cycloheximide, which prevents the RNA-directed synthesis of protein, are each effective in preventing the appearance of increased tyrosine hydroxylase after reserpine administration. Hence the reserpine is believed to induce synthesis of new tyrosine hydroxylase molecules.

It is believed that the induction of new enzyme occurs by a transsynaptic mechanism. Reserpine depletes the stored norepinephrine in nerve terminals. The loss of the transmitter would then result in the lack of an appropriate output signal, which would then be detected at some remote point in a neural feedback loop and lead to increased stimulation of the norepinephrine perikaryon. This transsynaptic event, repeated often enough, would then induce new enzyme synthesis. This hypothesis is supported by the observation that, when the preganglionic input fibers to the superior cervical ganglion are severed, reserpine is no longer effective in inducing new synthesis of tyrosine hydroxylase.

The quantity of active enzyme found in the human brain varies with the location studied. Putamen, caudate nucleus, and substantia nigra have the highest concentration, while cerebellum and cerebral cortex have the least. Significant changes occur with growth and aging. Tyrosine hydroxylase in the caudate decreases rapidly up to age 20 and then declines slowly throughout life. In contrast, there is a continuous increase of this enzyme in the substantia nigra throughout life.

The second enzymatic step in the formation of the biogenic amines requires the enzyme DOPA-decarboxylase, which removes the carboxyl group from dihydroxyphenylalanine, producing dihydroxyphenylethylamine, abbreviated as dopamine (DA). This enzyme is not specific to DOPA; it will decarboxylate other aromatic amino acids as well as 5-hydroxytryptophan (see below). The bulk of the enzyme is located in the cytoplasm of nerve terminals. In contrast to tyrosine hydroxylase, it is present in such great excess that, even after administration of inhibitors which reduce its activity to 5% of normal, no detectable change in dopamine or norepinephrine concentrations occurs. Thus under most conditions it is not rate limiting.

In dopaminergic nerve terminals the synthetic reaction sequence ends at this step. In others an additional enzyme, dopamine beta hydroxylase, adds an additional hydroxyl group to the side chain of the substrate. The product is norepinephrine (NE). All of these reactions also occur in peripheral nerve and in the adrenal medulla as well, where an additional enzymatic step adds a methyl group to NE, producing adrenalin. The activity of dopamine beta hydroxylase is dependent upon the presence of ionized copper in the cytoplasm; nutritional deficiencies or drugs such as disulfiram and its reduction product, diethyldithiocarbamate, which converts the copper to a nonionized form, result in a decreased conversion of tyrosine to NE and an increased accumulation of DA by inhibiting the final hydroxylation step.

DA and NE, synthesized in this manner in nerve terminals, are immediately taken up into storage granules. Amine molecules remaining in the cytoplasm are subject to the action of the mitochondrial enzyme, monoamine oxidase (MAO), which removes the amino group and converts biogenic amines to inactive products (see Figure 12-3). Thus MAO imposes another regulation on the amine transmitter content of nerve terminals; if excess synthesis occurs the unneeded amount, as defined by those molecules which have not been accepted into storage sites, is rapidly converted to aldehydes by MAO. Individual isoenzymes of MAO are known to have regional specificity in the brain. Thus the caudate nucleus contains an isoenzyme of MAO that is almost specific for DA and has little effect on other amines. Inhibitors of MAO will be discussed in Chapter 13.

The aldehydes are subject to further enzymatic conversion. The reductive pathway leads to formation of hydroxyl derivatives (alcohols) such as dihydroxyphenylglycol. The oxidative pathway, requiring the enzyme aldehyde dehydrogenase, yields the acid derivatives, such as dihydroxymandelic acid. Thus these substances, which are formed in the nerve terminal, represent the metabolism of excess DA and NE—in effect, the nonfunctional utilization of the amine transmitters.

Metabolites that are formed in the course of functional utilization have been identified. When NE is released by a nerve impulse from an active storage site in the nerve terminal, it moves across the synaptic cleft and activates a postsynaptic receptor. The receptor, after initiating a sequence of changes leading to a partial depolarization of the postsynaptic membrane, must then be restored to its initial state if it is to be responsive to another wave of NE molecules. Thus removal of NE is required, most of which is accomplished by diffusion back to the presynaptic membrane and re-uptake into the nerve terminal. A small amount that does not readily return is acted on by the enzyme catechol-O-

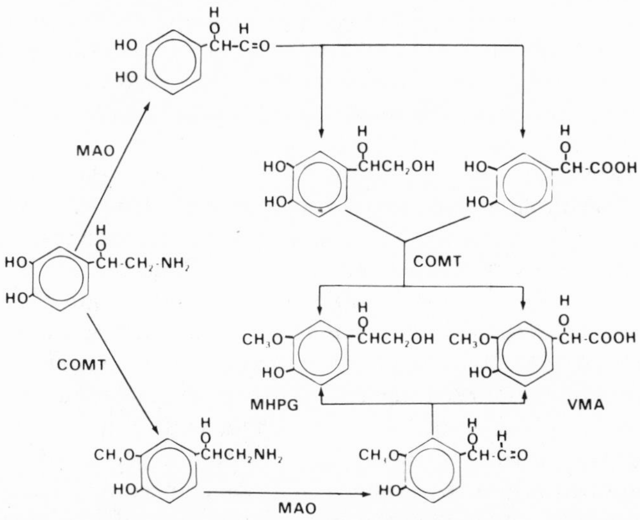

Figure 12-3. Metabolism of norephinephrine. Monoamine oxidase (MAO) and catechol-O-methyl transferase (COMT) are the major enzymes involved. Methoxyhydroxyphenylglycol (MHPG) and vanillylmandelic acid (VMA) are the end products.

methyl transferase (COMT) is the synaptic cleft (see Figure 12-3). The product, 3-O-methyl norepinephrine, also known as normetanephrine is inactive; 3-O-methyl dopamine is similarly formed from DA.

The amount of the O-methylated products formed is an indication of functional utilization of the transmitters, and the relative proportions of O-methylated products to acid metabolites are an index of functional to nonfunctional utilization of the biogenic amines. The index increases when the level of neural activity increases because the average amount of amine transmitter found in the synaptic cleft is increased in proportion to the frequency of nerve impulses.

The O-methylated proudcts are subject to further metabolism, first by MAO and then by reductive or oxidative enzymes. The final products from NE are vanillyl mandelic acid (VMA) and 3-methoxy, 4-hydroxyphenyl glycol (MHPG). These same substances are also obtained by the action of COMT on 3, 4-

dihydroxy phenyl glycol and 3, 4-dihydroxy mandelic acid. Thus the total amount of VMA and MHPG found represents the sum of functional and nonfunctional utilization. An analogous product, 4-hydroxy, 3-methoxy phenylacetic acid, known as homovanillic acid (HVA) is the end product of DA metabolism.

A shift in the ratio of functional to nonfunctional metabolites is demonstrable in animals after inhibition of MAO. Under such conditions there is a concomitant behavioral excitation. The apparent utility of MAO inhibitors in bringing about remission from depression in human subjects (described in more detail in Chapter 13) is thought to be based on similar changes. However, there is some evidence that the situation is more complicated. It has been suggested that the naturally occurring inhibitor of tyrosine hydroxylase is not NE, the synthetic end product, but 3, 4-dihydroxy phenyl acetaldehyde, a metabolite produced by the action of MAO on DA. Thus it might be conjectured that MAO inhibitors, by preventing the formation of the aldehyde needed for the feedback inhibition of tyrosine hydroxylase, not only allow an excess of NE and DA to accumulate but also promote the more rapid synthesis of these transmitters. Since it has been postulated that it is the newly synthesized NE that is preferentially released by a nerve impulse, MAO inhibitors may therefore cause the excessive production of easily releasable NE.

Some insight on the relation of amine transmitter utilization to behavioral states has been obtained from detailed studies of sleep cycles. Although a particular affective state is not to be inferred from sleep per se, there is a strong correlation between sleep disturbances and manic-depressive disease. In addition, it has been reported that drugs having antidepressive activity also decrease the proportion of the sleep cycle spent in REM sleep. Studies of the spontaneous neural activity of NE-containing neurons in the locus caeruleus of the cat have demonstrated that the rate of spontaneous discharge was low during sleep, except for that portion of the sleep cycle characterized as REM sleep. Additionally, it was found that spontaneous activity was low if the animal was awake and quiet, but it increased greatly during a period described as an attentive waking state. An increased discharge rate of these neurons implies a greater utilization of the transmitter, NE, at their terminals.

REM sleep is accompanied by characteristic fast activity in the EEG. The remaining portion of the sleep cycle is characterized by a much lower level of EEG activity and is designated as "slow wave" sleep (SS). The existence of SS is dependent upon another amine transmitter, serotonin. Most of the neurons containing serotonin are located in the raphe nuclei. When lesions are produced in these nuclei there is a loss of SS that is proportional to the extent of the lesion. A persistent insomnia resulted from lesions of 80% of the nuclei. The animals were constantly in motion and had an increased heart rate. Fast EEG activity was predominant. When the extent of the lesions did not exceed 50% of the nuclei, there was a partial recovery after 2 days of insomnia. Alteration of the brain serotonin content by administration of inhibitors of synthesis or metabolism was accompanied by increased SS when serotonin was elevated or decreased SS when serotonin synthesis was decreased.

Although the biosynthetic sequence that leads from the amino acid, tryptophan, to the transmitter, serotonin (Figure 12-2), and the tyrosine to the NE pathway are analogous, they differ from each other with respect to the biological and experimental means available for controlling the overall rate of synthesis.

The rate-limiting step in the sequence is the hydroxylation of tryptophan. However, in distinction to the hydroxylation of tyrosine which is rate limiting because of a relative deficiency of tyrosine hydroxylase, tryptophan hydroxylase is usually present in sufficient supply. Rather, it is the relative intracellular deficiency of the substrate, tryptophan, that causes this step to be rate limiting. Thus all factors that control the intraneuronal availability of tryptophan will ultimately reflect on cerebral synthesis of serotonin.

Control starts with dietary intake, since tryptophan is an essential amino acid. A significant portion is metabolized in the liver by the enzyme pyrrolase (see Chapter 8). Since the adrenocortiocosteroids increase liver pyrrolase activity they provide an indirect control of the quantity of tryptophan ultimately available to the CNS. That part of the dietary tryptophan that is not metabolized by the liver is transported by the plasma to the blood-brain barrier, where it must compete with tyrosine, phenylalanine, leucine, isoleucine, and valine for transport into the brain. Thus mere ingestion of high protein foods does not inevitably result in elevated brain tryptophan and serotonin; the determining factor is the ratio of tryptophan to the other neutral amino acids. Plasma tryptophan concentration is also dependent on insulin secretion; thus a high carbohydrate diet, which stimulates insulin secretion, will elevate plasma tryptophan and hence CNS tryptophan.

The movement of tryptophan from the blood capillaries to neurons probably occurs via glial cells. One research group has found that stimulation of serotonin synthesis leads to an increased rate of uptake of tryptophan from the blood as well as from the cerebrospinal fluid in experimental animals. Since increased serotonin synthesis implies increased neuronal demand, there appears to be a positive neural feedback loop operating, whereby tryptophan transport into the brain is increased to accommodate the requirement for additional serotonin production. These researchers have suggested that transport across the capillary-glial interface, and also across the glial-neuronal interface, requires cyclic AMP. They further suggest that NE, various drugs, and changes in the ionic environment might control cyclic AMP formation and hence regulate tryptophan transport and serotonin synthesis.

Tryptophan hydroxylase is found in particularly high concentrations in the subcellular particles of nerve terminals. This particle-bound tryptophan hydroxylase occurs in brain regions where the terminals of serotoninergic neurons are found, as well as in the raphe nuclei which contain most of the serotoninergic perikarya of the brain. Recently a soluble tryptophan hydroxylase has also been shown to occur in the same brain regions. The septal area is one of the sites containing a large number of serotoninergic terminals. Unlike regions such as the colliculus and hippocampus, which lose most of their tryptophan hydroxylase activity after administration of the inhibitor para chlorophenylalanine, the soluble tryptophan hydroxylase of the septal area is unaffected. These results, coupled with the observation that the soluble tryptophan hydroxylase activity is unaltered in the septal area, but reduced elsewhere after lesions of the perikarya of the raphe nuclei, and further coupled with the observation that such lesions reduce serotonin in all regions, suggest that the septal enzyme is not localized in nerve terminals. The researchers suggested that the results were compatible with the existence of an isoenzyme specific to the area and localized in other neural elements or perhaps in glial cells.

When the septal area, which is a part of the limbic system, is damaged by lesions in experimental animals, a state of viciousness and easily elicited rage occurs. The integrity of the area is apparently necessary to inhibit such behavior. Hence the presence of an unusually stable form of tryptophan hydroxylase would tend to promote the neurochemical stability of the area by synthesizing the serotonin needed for inhibitory activity, thus protecting the organism against surges of very inappropriate behavior. If these speculations are accepted as a basis for discussion, one more intriguing possibility exists: if a stable tryptophan hydroxylase is needed, there may be naturally occurring substances that will from time to time inhibit the less stable form of tryptophan hydroxylase in other brain areas, thus producing sporadic deficiencies in serotonin. Speculation about the behavioral consequences of such variations will be deferred to the following chapter.

The formation of serotonin from 5-hydroxytryptophan is catalyzed by a decarboxylase enzyme whose abundance and nonspecificity are such that it is not likely to be a control point in the biosynthesis of serotonin. Excess serotonin is converted to 5-hydroxy indole acetaldehyde by MAO (see Figure 12-4); further oxidation by an aldehyde dehydrogenase produces 5-hydroxyindole acetic acid (5-HIAA). Alternatively, the aldehyde can be reduced to 5-hydroxy tryptophol which in turn may acquire a methyl group with the aid of the enzyme hydroxyindole-O-methyl transferease (HIOMT). The product, 5-methoxy tryptophol, is found in high concentration in the pineal gland. Serotonin itself can be acetylated to produce N-acetyl serotonin; this substance when acted on by HIOMT is converted to melatonin. Although melatonin was first identified in the pineal gland, where its high concentration is subject to diurnal variation, it has recently been shown to be present in several regions of the CNS. Melatonin is known to be an indirect regulator of the menstrual cycle through its actions on the follicle-stimulating hormone (see Chapter 6); other actions in the CNS are presently under investigation.

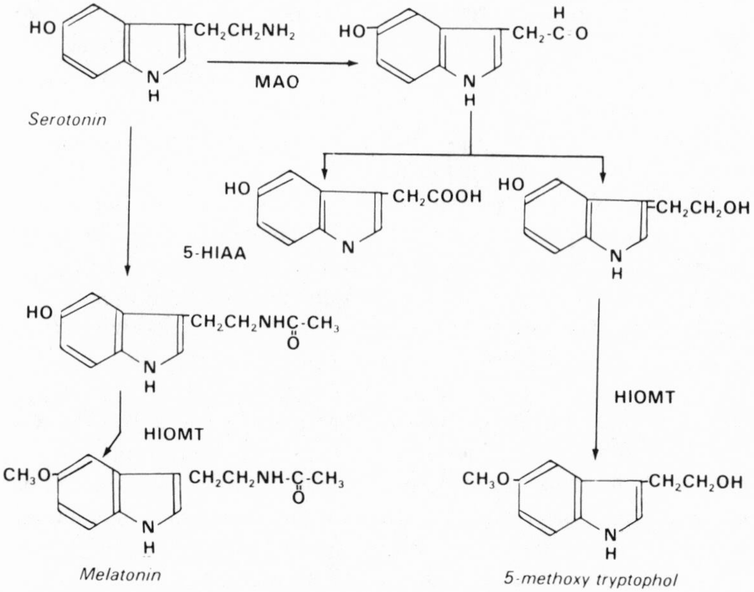

Figure 12-4. Metabolism of serotonin. Monoamine oxidase (MAO) and hydroxy indole-O-methyl transferase (HIOMT) are the principal enzymes. Hydroxyindole acetic acid (HIAA) is a major metabolite.

Steroid Hormones and Behavior

The close relation between affective state and the functioning of the adrenal cortex has been known for many years. The changes in affect in that condition of adrenocortical insufficiency known as Addison's disease were found by its discoverer to include inability to concentrate, drowsiness, restlessness, insomnia, irritability, and apprehension. Since that time it has been repeatedly observed that patients with Addison's disease are often depressed and occasionally euphoric. Similarly in Cushing's syndrome, which results in an increase in cortisol, it has been observed that the mental symptoms include either depression or mania. Since each of these diseases is accompanied by a variety of severe disturbances of peripheral physiology it is not possible to infer a direct causal relationship from these observations alone. However, it has been reported that corticosteroids administered for medical purposes sometimes produce depression, hypomania, or psychotic states that may include perceptual abnormalities, hallucinations, and depersonalization.

The corticosteroids (Figure 2-1) are known to have direct effects on neural responsivity. A computed measurement of the EEG, known as the average evoked potential, can be made by observing the EEG at some precisely reproducible time after a brief sensory input. Repetition of many such measurements leads to the calculation of a change in the average amplitude of the EEG, causally linked to the input signal. It has been found that cortisol decreases the amplitude of this average evoked potential. The result is consistent with the observation that the diurnal fluctuation in the corticosteroid concentration in the blood is related to changes in sensory threshold (see Chapter 6).

The various interactions of the corticosteroids with other neurochemical systems may result in control or modification of biogenic amine activity. Cortisol may exert indirect control over serotonin metabolism since an excess is known to induce the formation of tryptophan pyrrolase; as mentioned previously, this liver enzyme reduces the amount of tryptophan available to the plasma by diverting it to another metabolic pathway. More directly, it has been found that corticosterone can regulate the amount of tryptophan hydroxylase found in rat brain. Removal of the adrenal glands led to a large decrease in activity of the enzyme measured in the midbrain region. When adrenalectomized rats were resupplied with corticosterone the tryptophan hydroxylase levels rose toward normal. Since this restorative effect was blocked by the protein synthesis inhibitor, cyclohexidine, it was concluded that new synthesis of the enzyme was induced by corticosterone. The same researchers also observed that a stressful environment, known to elevate corticosterone levels, was accompanied by an increased tryptophan hydroxylase activity in the rat midbrain region.

Cortisol has been found to regulate the rate of uptake of NE from a nutrient solution, by slices of rat cerebral cortex. When the slices were incubated with cortisol and were then exposed to NE, they were able to accumulate increased amounts of the transmitter. It was demonstrated that the effect was dependent upon an amine "pump" which accumulated NE intracellularly against a concentration gradient. It is intriguing to consider the possibility that the reduction by cortisol of the average evoked potential as well as its ability to decrease sensitivity to sensory input may be related to this re-uptake phenomenon. If excess cortisol overactivates the amine pump, re-uptake may occur too soon to allow complete transmission of the informational content of each nerve impulse across the synapse, thereby producing a decreased level of neural functioning.

The relation between variations in the sex hormones and cyclic mood changes constitutes one of the clearest associations between endogenous chemistry and affect, particularly with respect to premenstrual mood changes. Depressed mood and irritability are common symptoms, arising 5 or more days prior to and continuing several days after menstruation. Estrogen secretion by a developing follicle is increased early in the cycle as a result of the action of the follicle-stimulating hormone; it continues after the induction of ovulation that is brought about by the luteinizing hormone. Progesterone secretion by the developing corpus luteum occurs during the postovulatory part of the cycle. Both hormones decrease rapidly a few days prior to menstruation. The phase of rising estrogen production has been correlated with a sense of well-being and an increased sex drive. It has been noted that the frequency of human intercourse is highest at ovulation. Androgens also increase libido in both men and women.

Two other naturally occurring conditions are also associated with an increased frequency of mood disturbance. During the period following childbirth there is a rapid fall in progesterone and estradiol, sometimes associated with a lowered mood or a mild depression. These postpartum depressions have their counterpart in the postmenopausal depressions which are also accompanied by estrogen depletion.

Whether both estrogens and progesterone are directly related to the changes in affect is a matter that is subject to ongoing research. With experimental animals it has been possible to show that the stimulus level necessary to produce an electroconvulsion (ECS) is decreased by estrogens and raised by progesterone, indicating some dissociation of actions of these hormones. Progesterone has also been found to have sedative and anaesthetic properties and to depress arousal mechanisms and cause a slowing of the EEG. Progesterone is suspected to be a factor in premenstrual mood disturbances since affective changes are said not to occur during anovulatory cycles; such cycles are character- ized by the presence of follicles which secrete estrogen and by the absence of progesterone secretion by the corpus luteum, since that structure only develops if ovulation occurs.

At the neurochemical level, there is an interesting interaction between progesterone and regulation of the transmitter amines. It has been reported that the enzymatic activity of the MAO isoenzymes in rat brain depends upon the degree of association with phospholipids; an enzyme devoid of phospholipids is almost totally inactive. It was found, by studying the subcellular distri- bution, that 80% of the brain progesterone is associated with MAO in the mitochondrial fraction. Since progesterone is a lipidlike substance, it seems possible that brain MAO activity might be altered by association with progesterone as well as with phospholipids. In accordance with this expectation it was observed that progesterone administration did increase MAO activity in rats.

Similarly, it was found that the MAO activity of the human endometrium increases tenfold by the 19th day of the menstrual cycle and returns to normal on the 23rd day; there is a suggested relation to progesterone secretion.

It is known that progesterone passes through the blood-brain barrier readily. Thus increased brain levels would be expected during the first 20 to 25 days of the menstrual cycle. If human brain MAO activity were altered by association with progeste- rone, there would be an increased enzyme activity up until a few days before menstruation, at which time a dramatic fall in enzyme activity might occur. It has already been mentioned that there are several forms of MAO, having differing substrate specificities, so that the effect of progesterone could be exerted equally on all forms or almost specifically on only one. Whether one or all species of MAO might be subject to activation by progesterone, the effect of rising or falling progesterone would be rising or falling MAO activity in the brain during the menstrual cycle. The foregoing discussion is based on the still unproved assumption that the probable effect of progesterone on rat brain MAO will also hold true for human brain. What follows is a speculation, anticipating that such proof will be obtained.

Enzyme induction is a general phenomenon. It is not unlikely that MAO will also be shown to be inducible and that its synthesis will be controlled by some negative feedback system that detects its level of functioning. Thus an MAO-progesterone association whose enzymatic activity is slowly increasing during the menstrual cycle may provide a signal to turn off further synthesis and thus stabilize the relation between MAO and the amine transmitter it helps to regulate. However, sudden withdrawal of the progesterone, with a concomitant decline in the level of MAO activity, may produce a signal to induce rapid synthesis of new enzyme. If a transient overproduction occurs, as is characteristic of such control systems, it may occasionally be of sufficient magnitude to seriously deplete the amine transmitter. To the extent that the amine hypothesis of affective state is valid, such an event would be translated into a rapid decline in the level of affect.

It is necessary to point out once again that these are only unsupported speculations at the present time. Such speculative discussions are introduced in an attempt to convey the sense of change and challenge that characterizes these fields of research. Previous chapters have described a small sample of the many solid facts available to researchers in the brain sciences. Some of these facts, as in the case of early postnatal imprinting of chemically modulated adult behavior, seem well matched to the problem at hand. Others, as in the discussion of mental illnesses to follow in the next chapter, have been remarkably successful in generating useful empirical therapies, but they fall far short of providing a viable theoretical structure upon which to base further therapeutic advances. Under such circumstances reasonable speculations temporarily serve as surrogate facts and thereby help to shape the quest for new knowledge.

13

Chemical Aspects of Mental Illness

DIAGNOSIS AND CLASSIFICATION of mental illness is always subject to disagreement among equally competent authorities. The difficulty is exemplified by the diagnostic term, "schizoaffective," which might be applied to a particular patient by one therapist while another will see the same patient as manic-depressive. Although each will describe the symptom cluster in similar terms, the significance assigned to various symptoms leads to the differing diagnosis and prognosis. Nevertheless, there are subgroups of patients who will be recognized by most diagnosticians as clearly belonging either to the schizophrenic group or to the manic-depressive group, based on the existence of some key symptoms as well as on the natural history of the disease. Similarly, it is possible to find a subgroup who is primarily afflicted with alcoholism. Relatively successful psychopharmacological treatments for many members of the manic-depressive group have been in existence for many years. In contrast, analogous treatments for schizophrenic subjects are less advanced and at present succeed at best in alleviating acute symptomatology. For the alcoholic patient there is at present no systematic chemotherapeutic treatment; exhortation, punishment, and aversive behavior modification are the only available modes of care. The neurochemical basis for present and emerging therapies of manic-depressive disease, the hypothesized neurochemical defects in the schizophrenias, and the present state of knowledge about the neurochemical correlates of alcoholism constitute the subject matter of this chapter.

Manic-Depressive Disease

It has been estimated that there are several million sufferers of this disease in the United States at the present time. The disease is subclassified according to the categories of bipolar and unipolar; the bipolar group is sometimes further differentiated according to whether the initial episode that was severe enough to require hospitalization was a manic or a depressive episode. Unipolar patients are those who have only depressive episodes. In all categories most patients have variable periods of normal functioning. Diagnosis requires that there be no other apparent cause for the mania or depression, that is, that a condition of primary affective disease exists.

Depressive episodes are usually characterized by feelings of hopelessness, guilt, low self-esteem, suicidal ideation or overt suicide attempts, a lethargy termed "psychomotor retardation" or an uncontrollable agitation and restlessness, inability to concentrate, decreased sex drive, sleep disturbance, and poor appetite. Less frequently, obsessive guilt merging with paranoid ideation may be present. Hypomanic episodes are characterized by pressured speech, a "flight of ideas," inappropriate handling of financial matters, grandiosity, hypersexuality, and a much reduced sleep cycle. The fully manic individual may in addition be exceedingly disruptive and assaultive; both the manic and the hypomanic are easily distracted.

Depressive episodes of manic-depressive disease usually last for several weeks to several months; occasionally a chronic depression, lasting for years, may occur. Hypomanic episodes are generally shorter in duration, partially because the socially unacceptable behavior of the hypomanic patient leads to prompt treatment. Occasionally, a patient will be found who is described as a rapid cycler, having several episodes of mania and depression each year. More rarely, a patient can be observed to "switch" from extreme dejection to inappropriate elation over a period of minutes.

Psychopharmacological treatment of manic-depressive disease developed along with the growth of the biogenic amine hypothesis. There had been a background of experience with the use of reserpine as an antihypertensive agent; tranquilization was a common side effect. Additionally, there were reports that depression sometimes followed its use. These were soon followed by research studies demonstrating that increased excretion of serotonin metabolites accompanied the ingestion of reserpine. Soon thereafter observations with experimental animals demonstrated that the serotonin concentration in the brain was decreased by reserpine. At about the same time it was noted that iproniazid, a substance employed for the chemotherapeutic treatment of tuberculosis, produced an excited state in some patients. When iproniazid was found to be an MAO inhibitor, and to elevate serotonin levels in animal brains, the outlines of the biogenic amine hypothesis began to emerge: reserpine depleted brain serotonin and caused depression, while iproniazid elevated brain serotonin and caused behavioral excitation. It was soon observed that similar changes in brain norepinephrine occurred with these agents. Many drugs were then synthesized and tested for the ability to alter brain biogenic amine levels. Several of those that elevated the amine levels were found to have antidepressant activity in clinical populations.

Antidepressant Drugs

The chemical structures of several categories of antidepressant drugs are depicted in Figure 13-1. The fact that they are antidepressants, coupled with the observations that they alter amine transmitter levels and metabolism, constitutes the major portion of the evidence for the biogenic amine hypothesis of affective state.

Administration of monoamine oxidase inhibitors such as phenelzine, nialamide, and tranylcypromine leads immediately to evidence for an increase in the amine transmitter content of both peripheral and CNS synapses. The peripheral effects, easily ob-

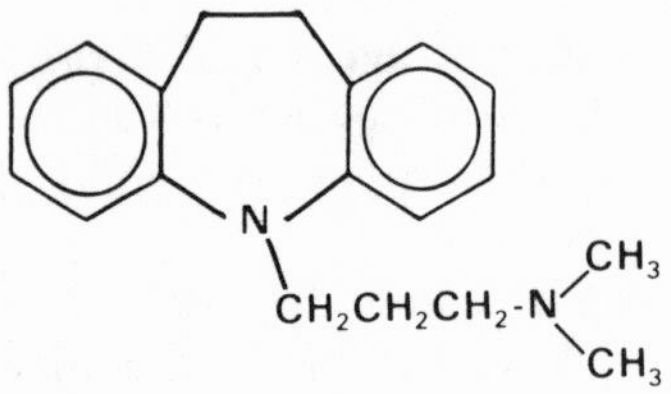

Imipramine (Tofranil)

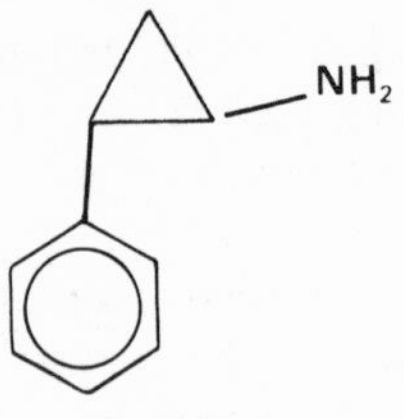

Tranylcypromine (Parnate)

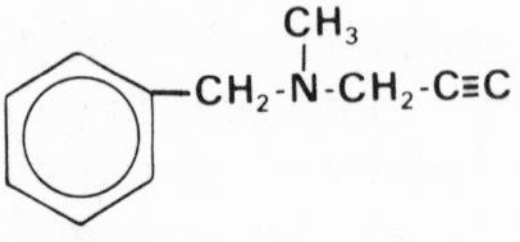

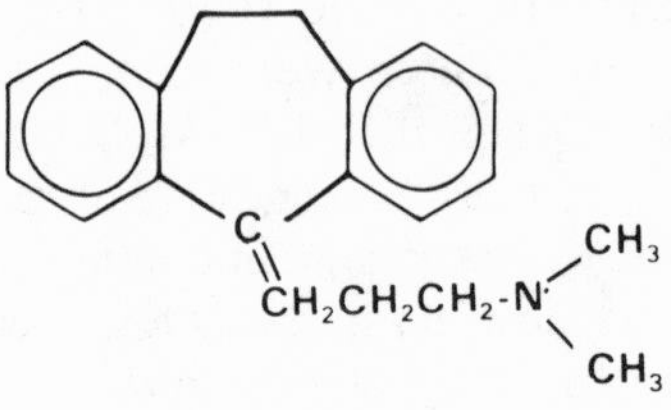

Amitriptylene (Elavil)

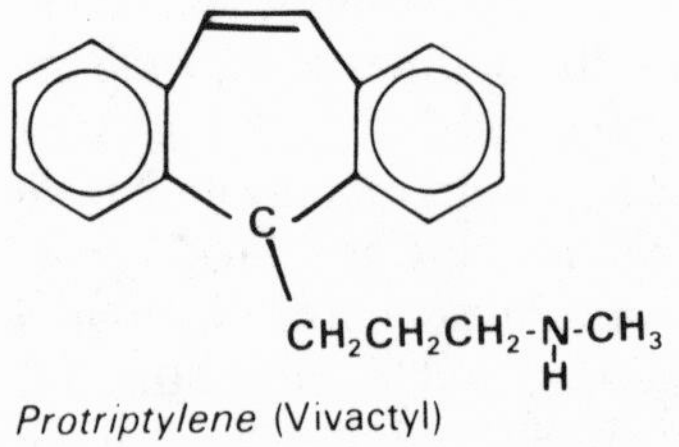

Pargyline

Protriptylene (Vivactyl)

Figure 13-1. Structures of some antidepressants.

served after administration to human subjects, depend on the increase in activity of the sympathetic nervous system with consequent overbalancing of the parasympathetic effects. (See Chapter 11 for more details of the counterbalancing actions of these two components of the autonomic nervous system.) Monoamine oxidase inhibitors appear to simulate ganglionic blocking agents, and they may produce orthostatic hypotension, blurred vision, dry mouth, constipation, and impotence, among other symptoms.

Biochemical evidence that the monoamine oxidase inhibitors increase amine transmitter levels in human subjects has depended upon measured changes in the quantities of amine transmitter metabolites found in the urine, blood, and CSF. Monoamine oxidase inhibitors combine irreversibly with monoamine oxidase (MAO) and inhibit the enzyme activity for several days, until more enzyme is synthesized. Since there are several MAO isoenzymes present in the brain it would be desirable to know if some of the various inhibitors act preferentially against a specific isoenzyme. The question of specificity has also been directed at the possibility that the MAO inhibitors inhibit the re-uptake mechanism for amine transmitters. It is clear, however, that whether or not the re-uptake mechanism is also involved in their actions, a principal effect of MAO inhibitors is to increase the concentration of the biogenic amines. When combined with other agents that produce a further increase in the biogenic amines, hypertension and other serious side effects are likely to occur. It is customary to caution patients receiving MAO inhibitors not to consume aged cheeses, chicken livers, wine, and certain other foods because the tyramine that they contain, accumulating in the absence of active MAO molecules, can displace NE from nerve terminals, thereby producing hypertension and other side effects when the target neurons are part of the sympathetic peripheral system. Some MAO inhibitors cause hypotension; it has been hypothesized that this is due to the increased concentration of "false" transmitters such as para hydroxy phenylethanolamine, which effectively block the normal actions of NE and adrenaline.

There is a large group of synthetic substances composed of three fused rings and containing various substituents. These tricyclic antidepressants (Figure 13-1) have been shown to block the re-uptake of some of the amine transmitters from the synaptic cleft, thereby increasing their effective concentration (see Chapter 12). When this process was studied in detail in slices of rat brain it was found that the tricyclics appeared to compete with the transmitters for sites on the "amine pump." A comparison of short- versus long-term effects of imipramine on NE metabolism in the rat brain indicated that a single dose of the drug inhibited both the uptake and the metabolism of NE; in contrast when imipramine was injected over a 3-week period the uptake of NE was inhibited as with the single dose, but the functional metabolism was accelerated, as evidenced by an increase in normetanephrine and a decrease in deaminated metabolites. Since an antidepressant effect of the tricyclics requires 1 to 3 weeks to develop, these observations on the rat brain may be significantly related to the events occurring in the human brain.

When depressed patients were treated with tricyclic drugs it was found that the quantity of the NE metabolite, 3-methoxy, 4-hydroxy mandelic acid (see Chapter 12), excreted in the urine was decreased only during the period of administration of the drug. This is evidence that NE metabolism in humans is altered in the same direction as in rats by these substances.

Further evidence for the relation of the amine transmitters to affective state comes from studies of their normal metabolism, unaltered by drugs. It has been reported that the CSF concentration of 3-methoxy, 4-hydroxy phenyl glycol (MHPG), a metabolite that reflects total utilization of NE (see Chapter 12), is lower in depressed patients than in controls or manic patients. These observations were consistent with earlier studies which showed that similar changes occurred in urinary MHPG. However, since the metabolite appearing in the CSF reflects brain and spinal cord NE metabolism, while urinary MHPG is indicative of total body NE metabolism, the CSF studies added strong support to the postulate that changes in NE metabolism are correlated with affective state.

The most reliable treatment of depression, in the sense that remission of symptoms is obtained, is electroconvulsive therapy (ECT). As with other treatment modalities, repeated ECT is required before therapeutic effects become apparent. Many studies of the effects of repeated ECT on animals have been performed with a view toward detecting neurochemical changes that might reveal the mechanisms involved. One of these has demonstrated that after application of a single electroconvulsive shock (ECS) to rats, the rate of uptake of radioactively labeled NE by portions of cerebral cortex was markedly diminished; the data were interpreted to mean that NE would reside for a longer time in the synaptic cleft rather than become deactivated by reaccumulation into the presynaptic terminal. The altered rate of re-uptake was no longer apparent 18 hours after the single ECS. However, repeated ECSs led to a sustained decrease in the re-uptake rate. These results therefore suggest that ECT functions at least in part by altering NE distribution in the brain, with the result that the

NE functionally available to the synaptic cleft is increased. Other researchers have shown that functional utilization of NE (see Chapter 12) is increased by ECS. A general picture emerges indicating that affective states and affect-altering drugs correlate with increased functional utilization of NE.

Antimanic Drugs

Mania, the other pole of bipolar affective disease, has been controlled with a wide variety of tranquilizing agents (Figure 13-2), among which the phenothiazines, thioxanthenes, and butyrophenones are prominent. These substances, known as neuroleptics or major tranquilizers, have been shown to inhibit postsynaptic receptors. By blocking these sites they make it less possible for a transmitter, released into the synaptic cleft, to depolarize the next neuron and thus initiate a nerve impulse. In some instances the reduced impulse flow causes a neurochemical activation of a neuronal feedback loop. For example, some afferent dopaminergic fibers from the striatum provide a feedback signal to the substantia nigra which controls the firing rate of the nigral fibers. An increased formation and release of DA results from use of the neuroleptic; however, the DA is still ineffective because of the blocked postsynaptic receptor. Recently it has been shown that the increased firing rate leads to a conformational change in the tyrosine hydroxylase molecule; the enzyme becomes more responsive to its substrate and less affected by the feedback inhibition caused by the product.

DA is thought to act on some postsynaptic membranes by activating the enzyme adenyl cyclase; this enzyme catalyzes the cyclization of adenosine monophosphate to cyclic adenosine monophosphate (cAMP). Fluphenazine, a phenothiazine, has been found to be a competitive inhibitor of adenyl cyclase. It appears that there are several varieties of adenyl cyclase having differing specificities for various hormones; in many peripheral tissues a catacholamine-sensitive adenyl cyclase system has properties typical of a beta adrenergic receptor. Adenyl cyclase activity and cAMP exist in higher concentration in the brain than in any other organ. The activation of the brain enzyme by catecholamines is dependent upon a narrow range of calcium ion concentration.

At least two adenyl cyclases occur in the brain; one in the

cerebellum is responsive to NE, while the other in the striatum is sensitive to DA. The properties of the DA-sensitive adenyl cyclase of the brain, which have been studied extensively, are such that it appears to be distinct from either the alpha or the beta adrenergic system. It is this particular adenyl cyclase that is strongly inhibited by fluphenazine and flupenthixol (Figure 13-2) and only weakly inhibited by chlorpromazine and haloperidol.

It is also possible that these drugs, which are employed not only to control mania but more importantly as general antipsychotic agents, act on specialized regions of the presynaptic membrane. Such regions are thought of as presynaptic receptors and may have a role in regulating transmitter release from the nerve terminal. The butyrophenones appear to block the impulse-induced release of DA from nerve terminals.

Evidence that cAMP metabolism is important in manic-depressive disease was obtained by a study of the urinary excretion of cAMP during the switch from depression to mania. In a group of patients who switched rapidly it was found that a transient increase in excretion of cAMP occurred just prior to the onset of the manic attack. The researchers suggested that cAMP was associated with a "trigger" for the switch.

The group of antipsychotic drugs illustrated in Figure 13-2 has a broad range of behavioral effects; among these are control of manic and hypomanic behavior. In contrast, lithium salts have apparently specific antimanic activity. Lithium is a trace element in nature, belonging to the Group I cations of the periodic table; the other members of Group I are sodium, potassium, rubidium, cesium, and franconium.

The antimanic properties of lithium were discovered serendipitously in 1949; since then several careful studies have demonstrated that its use results in a success rate of 80% when tested on a carefully defined population of manic-depressive subjects. In contrast to the antipsychotic agents which act almost immediately, lithium dosage for 5 to 10 days is required before its effects become apparent. Thus severely manic patients are usually treated initially with the neuroleptics and then with lithium. The result of continued treatment with lithium is reported to be superior to that of the neuroleptics, in that the patients feel normal rather than drugged. Moreover, mainten-

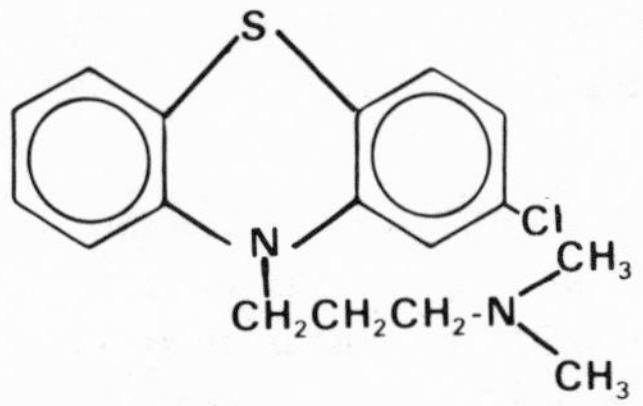

Chlorpromazine

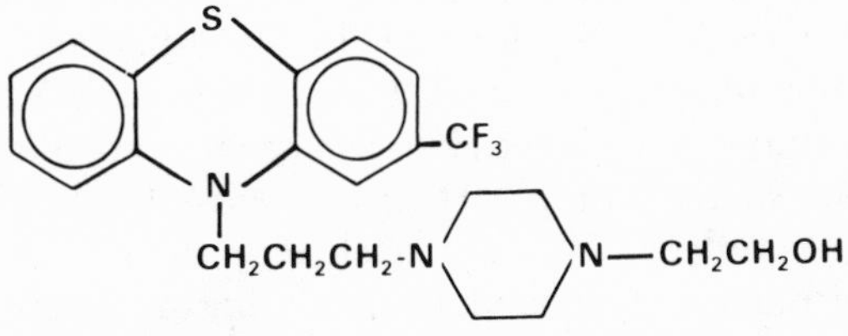

Fluphenazine

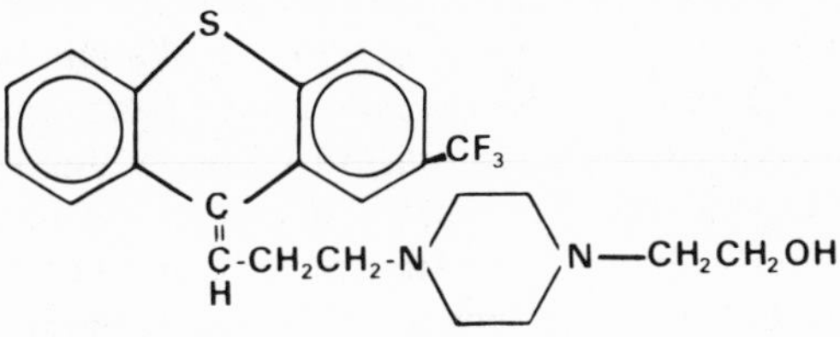

Flupenthixol

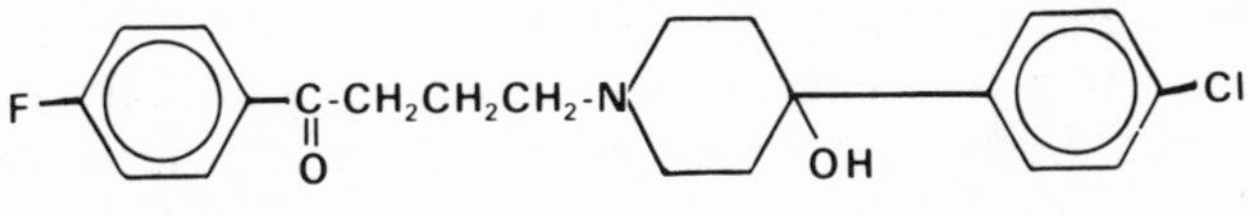

Haloperidol

Figure 13-2. Structures of some antipsychotic drugs.

ance therapy has been continued for many years with medically appropriate patients, using control measurements of blood lithium levels, without undesirable side effects. Patients experience a full range of emotions, intellectual activity, and unimpaired sex drive. The cyclic manic-depressive patient obtains significant prophylactic effect from lithium therapy, in that both manic and depressive episodes are much reduced in frequency and severity.

The neurochemical effects of lithium have been studied extensively. Some of the results are consistent with the biogenic amine hypothesis. A detailed study of the urinary excretion of NE, adrenaline, and their metabolites in a group of hypomanic patients revealed that lithium therapy was accompanied by a decreased excretion of normetanephrine and metanephrine, regardless of the therapeutic outcome. In those patients who responded to lithium, it was found that excretion of VMA and MHPG (see Chapter 12) decreased during remission. Since, of all the substances studied, only MHPG can cross the blood-brain barrier and thus reflect CNS neurochemistry, the results demonstrate that peripheral catecholamine metabolitism is decreased by lithium; it is reasonable to surmise that similar changes occur in the CNS.

For more specific information about the effects of lithium it is necessary to conduct studies in experimental animals. Isotopic tracer techniques were employed in an investigation that demonstrated a diversion of NE metabolism to the nonfunctional pathways (see Chapter 12) after either acute or chronic administration of lithium. It increased the rate of uptake of NE into synaptosomes and led to a decrease in normetanephrine and an increase in deaminated metabolites.

Although the results just cited would seem to include lithium within the field of the catecholamine hypothesis, there are many other known biochemical and neurophysiological effects of this ion. It has been reported to produce slowing of the human EEG and to shorten the duration of the action potential in preparations of isolated nerve, under experimental conditions where the sodium content of the normal medium is completely replaced by lithium. It has also been reported to decrease the conduction velocity measured in human nerves. Administered chronically to cats, it altered the sleep cycle so as to produce more slow wave and less REM sleep.

At the molecular level, lithium has been found to activate ATPase, the enzyme system implicated in the functioning of the sodium pump. When lithium-containing solutions were flowed over isolated nerves, the ATPase activity was increased. However, when the same nerves were stimulated, ATPase activity markedly diminished. If such results occurred in intact brain the nerve fibers would not be capable of sustaining normal functioning. After chronic lithium administration to rats, brain cAMP content was decreased. In contrast, the antidepressant drug desmethyl imipramine increased brain cAMP. These results could not be observed after acute ingestion. The researchers suggested that the therapeutic effect of lithium, known to occur only after chronic intake, might be due to decreased brain cAMP.

Lithium also has some generalized metabolic effects. It increased glucose uptake by rat brain and anaerobic metabolism at the expense of aerobic metabolism, as evidenced by an increased formation of lactate from glucose and a decreased formation of glutamate.

Deficits in the Amine Hypothesis

The observed effects of the antidepressant and antimanic agents are consistent with the biogenic amine hypothesis. Although the hypothesis cannot be considered proven by this array of observations, it is clear that neural pathways utilizing amines are closely involved in the variation of affective behavior. Hypotheses generate expectations: if a particular drug response occurs, then another agent, known to be involved in the same neurochemical sequence, should produce predictable clinical responses. The testing of hypotheses of this kind has recently led to the view that the amine hypothesis, although useful, has serious inadequacies.

The present state of the biogenic amine hypothesis suggests that, although the functional excess or deficit of NE leads to mania or depression, respectively, these behaviors only occur if serotonin metabolism is simultaneously deficient. That is, a lack of serotonin is a required condition for the expression of either pole of manic-depressive disease. If this is so, it should be possible to treat manic-depressive disease by increasing the brain serotonin content. It is known that brain serotonin synthesis is increased by selectively increasing the tryptophan content of the blood plasma, thereby increasing brain tryptophan and the activity of brain tryptophan hydroxylase (see Chapter 12).

When a group of depressed patients was treated by oral ingestion of repeated doses of 1-tryptophan, it was found by studying the cerebrospinal fluid concentration of the serotonin metabolite, 5HIAA, that serotonin synthesis and metabolism was increased as a result of the tryptophan administration. However, no therapeutic result was obtained. Since it was possible that a depression, once established, required simultaneous reversal of both the underlying serotonin deficit and the periodic catecholamine deficit, a further test was undertaken. Another group of depressed patients was treated with a combined dosage of L-tryptophan and L-DOPA; it was reasonably expected that L-DOPA, known to penetrate the blood-brain barrier, would be converted to DA at the same time that tryptophan increased serotonin metabolism. Once again no antidepressant response was obtained. Many of the same patients subsequently showed good responses to MAO inhibitors or to tricyclic antidepressants.

Other research groups have had similar results, or equivocal success with L-tryptophan. Since 5-hydroxy tryptophan is a more immediate precursor of serotonin, experimental administration of this substance to depressed patients was also investigated. Again the results were equivocal or negative. Analogous tests were conducted employing inhibitors of catecholamine synthesis with manic patients. Alpha methyl tryosine is an inhibitor of tyrosine hydroxylase, and its use should result in a deficit of NE and DA. Similarly, fusaric acid is an inhibitor of dopamine beta hydroxylase, and its use should result in a selective decrease in NE in the brain. The results of administration of either of these substances to manic patients were equivocal or negative.

These recent experimental investigations bring into question the validity of the amine hypothesis as a basis for generating further treatments of manic-depressive disease. There is therefore renewed interest in alternate hypotheses.

Electrolytes and Manic-Depressive Disease

Movement of the monovalent ions across axonal and post-synaptic membranes is inseparably related to the transfer of information within the CNS (see Chapter 8). Additionally, calcium ions are required for activation of several enzymes, including adenyl cyclase (see above), and magnesium ions are necessary for the functioning of ATPase, as well as for glycolytic and other enzymes. Thus the content of electrolytes within the periphery, reflecting to some extent at least brain electrolyte content, has received much theoretical and experimental attention.

Several researchers have suggested that there is a decrease in the total exchangeable sodium present in the body following recovery from depression. Exchangeable sodium is defined as that portion of the total body sodium, usually about 80%, that comes into equilibrium with radioactive sodium atoms within 24 hours. The magnitude of the reported changes is generally less than 10%, and it is sometimes so small as to be of questionable experimental validity. Since it has also been found that a sodium excretion, in excess of intake, occurs during the first day after lithium ingestion, it is not likely that these changes are causally related to the state of affect.

There is even less evidence presently available to support the postulate that total body potassium is decreased during the depressive state, although such results have been claimed. Calcium and magnesium levels in the blood have been studied in the several phases of manic-depressive disease. Once again there is no evidence of any consistent change correlated with affective state.

Thus, although the suspicion remains that electrolytes are intimately involved in changes in affective state, studies of whole-body electrolyte composition have not illuminated the problem. Attention has therefore turned to studies that can more precisely describe the compartmentalization of the various electrolytes and the means for regulating interchange between compartments, in the hope that the biochemical regulation of peripheral electrolyte distribution will have counterparts in CNS chemistry. A recent report indicates that the ATPase of red blood cell membranes, which has qualitative similarity to neuronal ATPase, may function differently as affective state changes. The researchers found that the portion of the ATPase activity identified with the sodium pump increased with improvement of mood in a group of depressive patients. The result of such changes would be to reduce the intracellular sodium concentration. Such an effect, occurring in neurons, would hyperpolarize the membranes. The result would be a nerve impulse that is less easily generated, but of greater electrical potential once formed.

Recently a new hypothesis of affective state has been proposed, based upon some ongoing experimental studies of the possible therapeutic potential of rubidium, another of the Group I cations. It has been reported that rubidium increased motor activity of rats and mice, augmented aggressive behavior, and activated the EEG of experimental animals and human subjects. Chronic administration to rats led to an increase in the functional utilization of NE. At the molecular level rubidium was found to decrease ATPase activity and to interfere with the accumulation of sodium and potassium by components of neuronal membranes. Considering that in every respect the known actions of rubidium are dissimilar, in a sense "opposite," to those of lithium and that lithium has proven antimanic activity, it was reasonable to test rubidium for antidepressive activity. At the present time the results of such tests are still inconclusive; some depressed patients have improved markedly during rubidium therapy, but the total number of cases studied is still too small to warrant a definite conclusion.

Although it would seem possible to include rubidium effects within the amine hypothesis, based on the changes in NE metabolism observed in rat brain, careful consideration of all of the data leads to an alternate hypothesis. Rubidium moves through membranes more slowly than does potassium, an ion with which it has marked qualitative correspondence. Lithium accelerates the movement of rubidium, and also probably that of potassium, through membranes. It has therefore been suggested that the effect of each of these ions is directed principally at neuronal membranes, particularly at axonal membranes. The time during which an action potential exists is dependent upon movement of sodium into the axoplasm and subsequent movement of potassium outward (see Chapter 8). If the slower moving rubidium ion partially replaces potassium the action potential will be extended in duration. Conversely, if lithium accelerates potassium movement the action potential will be contracted in duration. A longer lasting action potential would be considered to have more energy, resulting in an increased transmitter release when it reaches the synaptic terminal. The shorter action potential would result in diminished transmitter release. Thus transmission would depend on the shape of the action potential.

It is known that extended action potentials occur in isolated nerves in the presence of rubidium and that such preparations show contracted action potentials in the presence of lithium. It is therefore hypothesized that the behavioral effects of these ions are expressed through changes in the action potential and that in manic-depressive disease deficiencies in some membranes occur such that outward transport of potassium is retarded in the manic state and accelerated in the depressive state. Since this hypothesis has only recently been proposed, it is not possible at this time to guess at what its effect might be in furthering the generation of new information.

Schizophrenia

Although diagnosis of this disease, or this group of diseases, is very much dependent upon the psychiatric orientation of the diagnostician, certain features are common to most patients diagnosed as schizophrenic. These include the following: a chronic illness with no sustained intervals of normal functioning; flat affect; delusions or hallucinations, usually auditory in character; disorganized thought processes; poor social adjustment, sometimes described as autism; onset of the illness early in life, usually before age 40; a history of schizophrenia in the family; and the absence of other illnesses that might produce some of the same symptoms.

The present view is that schizophrenia, so defined, involves a significant disruption in dopaminergic systems in the CNS. The evidence for this is inferential as it is based in large part on the mode of action of the neuroleptics as well as on the implications of amphetamine-induced psychotic states. Phenothiazines, thioxanthenes, and butyrophenones (Figure 13-2) have proved particularly useful in controlling schizophrenic symptoms, allowing treatment outside of a hospital setting.

The neuroleptics that have the most potent antipsychotic effects are also likely to produce Parkinsonian symptoms as a side effect. Parkinson's disease is manifested by malfunction of the extrapyramidal system (see Chapter 1), as indicated by tremors and faulty control when gross muscle movements are required. This effect has been shown to be caused by a loss of dopaminergic neurons in the substantia nigra, and it can often be treated successfully with L-DOPA, the amino acid precursor of DA. Extra-pyramidal side effects are therefore considered to be an indication of interference with dopaminergic synapses. Since larger than normal amounts of methylated derivatives of DA, produced in the synaptic cleft, occur after phenothiazine and haloperidol administration, it is a reasonable conclusion that the interference with DA transmission involves not the release mechanism but rather the postsynaptic receptors. The inability of DA to stimulate the receptors is thought to lead to continued functioning of a neural feedback loop which produces an increased firing rate of the presynaptic neurons, leading to increased DA release and therefore increased methylation.

Some of the most effective butyrophenones are almost specific for dopaminergic systems, having almost no effect on NE. Adenyl cyclase (see above) is believed to be associated with the train of events in the postsynaptic membrane that leads through cAMP and subsequent phosphorylation of a membrane-bound protein to depolarization of the membrane. Adenyl cyclases exist throughout the body and have specific sensitivity to various hormones. A dopamine-sensitive adenyl cyclase is known to exist in the caudate nucleus, which contains the terminals of many dopaminergic fibers. This particular enzyme has been shown to be inhibited only by those phenothiazines and butyrophenones that are clinically effective.

The extensive animal experimentation with the isomers of amphetamine, outlined in Chapter 11, demonstrated that psychomotor activities were associated with NE release by amphetamine, and stereotypy with DA release. It was noted that the d isomer, Dexedrine, was 10 times more effective than the l-amphetamine, in producing psychomotor activity. In contrast, both Dexedrine and l-amphetamine were equally effective in producing stereotypy. When it was subsequently observed that Dexedrine and l-amphetamine are equally effective in producing psychotic states, it was inferred that dopaminergic systems are involved in psychosis. It has been reported that stereotypy in humans always accompanies amphetamine psychosis and does not occur in users who do not become psychotic.

There is thus a convergence of inferences based on the behavioral and neurochemical effects of the neuroleptics on the one hand, and amphetamine psychoses on the other. The neuro-leptics block DA receptors and alleviate schizophrenic symptomatology; amphetamine release of DA is associated with the development of psychotic states in normals and exacerbation of symptoms in schizophrenics. Studies of the brains of chronic schizophrenics, although not yet confirmed by other researchers, have provided some support for the hypothesis. It was found that the enzyme dopamine beta hydroxylase (DBH), which converts DA to NE, was present in varying, but lower, quantities in the pons, medulla, diencephalon, and hippocampus of the schizophrenic brains when compared with normals. The physical affinity of DBH for its substrate was similar in schizophrenic and normal brains, and it was also similar to the DBH obtained from normal human blood.

Less DBH might mean less NE and more DA are synthesized, consistent with the hypothesis that excess DA is associated with schizophrenia. However, it should be recalled that the current concepts of the neurochemical organization of the brain hold that only one transmitter exists in all of the axonal branches of any one neuron, so that a deficiency of DBH in NE-containing neurons should lead only to a NE deficit in those neurons, not to a DA excess. The authors of this study speculated that the schizophrenic disease process led to a destruction of NE terminals, and hence to the observed DBH loss. They concluded that the disease symptomatology was due to the NE deficit.

Although their interpretation might be correct, it is at variance with the body of work cited above which implicates DA in the psychotic state. A more speculative interpretation, with no present supporting evidence, is intriguing to consider. If the DBH deficit occurs in intact noradrenergic neurons, then the axonal branches and terminals of such neurons, normally "connected" to convey information via the transmitter NE, would in effect become converted to dopaminergic neurons, since the other part of the biosynthetic chain is unimpaired. Thus postsynaptic membranes which had been organized since birth to receive NE "messages" would, with the onset of the DBH deficit, begin to receive DA "messages," of different informational import. It is easy to imagine that the resulting confusion would be associated with a prevalent psychotic state.

There are alternate hypotheses of the schizophrenic state. The possibility that "false transmitters" and naturally occurring psychotomimetic agents are synthesized in small quantities in the normal state and in larger quantities in disease states has continued to receive experimental attention. Some support for the natural psychotomimetic hypothesis comes from observations on the effects of various amino acids on schizophrenic symptoms.

Although most of the amino acids tested were found to be without effect, methionine exacerbated the symptoms. This amino acid, via its derivative S-adenosylmethionine (SAM), is involved in the biochemical system that transfers methyl groups. Methylated derivatives of dopamine, serotonin, and norepinephrine (see Figure 13-3) could be produced in excess by vigor-

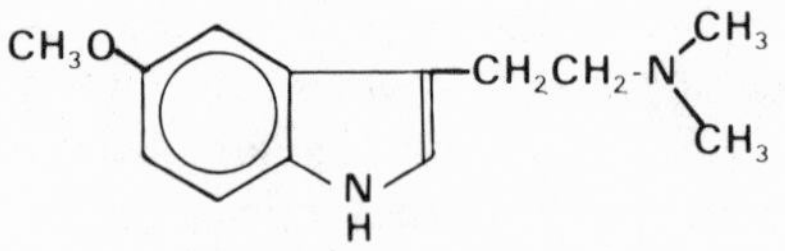

5-methoxydimethyl tryptamine

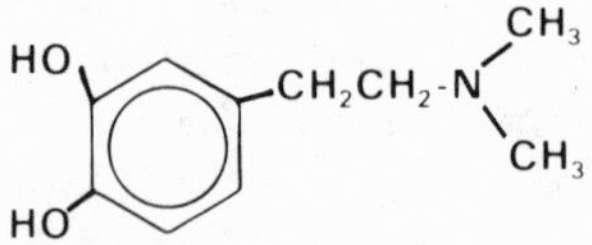

Dimethyl dopamine

Figure 13-3. Structures of methylated substances which may have psychotomimetic activity.

ous methylating systems. However, since the SAM-transfer enzyme has not as yet been demonstrated to occur in the brain, SAM is an unlikely methyl donor. More likely as a methyl donor is 5-methyl tetrahydrofolic acid (MTHF), which is utilized by brain tissue to form the potent psychotomimetic substance, 5-methoxydimethyl tryptamine (Figure 13-3). At the present time there are no data that would confirm or deny an increase in methylating processes in the psychotic states.

Alcoholism

The diagnostic criteria for this disease include physical manifestations of addiction and indications of CNS disturbance, as well as the usual signs of social deterioration. Addiction is apparent when the subject is unable to stop drinking or engages in elaborate maneuvers to control drinking, or by the occurrence of withdrawal symptoms such as tremors, convulsions, hallucinations, or delirium. CNS disturbances include blackouts as well as long-term consequences of alcoholism such as the Wernicke-Korsakoff syndrome. Social consequences in general involve a default of obligations; they may be evidenced by alcohol-related loss of employment, arrests for fighting or traffic offenses subsequent to alcohol intake, and loss of friends or family.

Alcoholism may be manifested either as chronic or episodic ingestion of excessive amounts; an excess is defined by the occurrance of at least some of the diagnostic criteria listed above. Research in this field has been directed toward two broad areas: identification of neurophysiological and neurochemical correlates of alcohol intake; and a description of those changes that are associated with chronic intake.

Neurobiological Effects of Ethyl Alcohol

Since the usual mode of alcohol input is by ingestion of solutions in concentrations of less than 50%, the first possible site of action is the gastrointestinal tract. It has been found that a 15% ethanol solution altered the patterns of absorption of amino acids from the intestine. Normally a few amino acids such as isoleucine, arginine, and methionine are more rapidly absorbed, and others such as glycine and glutamic acid are less rapidly absorbed than the average in a mixture of 18 common amino acids. The ingestion of ethyl alcohol resulted in a leveling of the pattern, with decreased absorption of the first group and increased absorption of the second group.

Ethanol itself is rapidly transferred between the blood and other tissues. A steady-state distribution between the blood and brain was found to occur in less than 2 minutes. It apparently distributes into all aqueous spaces in the body. Only a small portion is lost by excretion via the breath, sweat, and urine. Over 90% is metabolized at rates ranging from 100 to 200 milligrams each hour for each kilogram of body weight in humans.

Ethanol and a few other aliphatic alcohols have been shown to accumulate in biological membranes. They enter the lipid component of the membrane, expanding it at lower concentrations, and finally causing disorganization and disruption at much higher concentrations. At relatively high concentrations (2%) ethanol has been found to produce large changes in the action potential. The inward movement of sodium, associated with the rising phase of the action potential (see Chapter 8), is reduced while the falling phase is normal. Since this effect is enhanced by phospholipase A, an enzyme that removes a fatty acid moiety from phospholipids in the membrane, it seems likely that the altered action potential is due to an ethanol-lipid interaction. These observations, first made on the giant axon of the squid, were later extended to nerve fibers of the cat, rabbit, and frog. In all cases the action potentials were reduced in height and duration. An analogous decrease in excitability of frog skeletal muscle was produced by 1% ethanol. The high ethanol concentration employed in these experiments makes comparison with human usage of ethanol difficult; however, there are some other results at much lower concentrations that are more directly applicable.

There is a region of the lateral hypothalamus whose neurons appear to regulate eating and drinking behavior. Some of them are sensitive to the glucose concentration outside of the neuron, whereas others respond to the extracellular sodium concentration. A higher than normal concentration of sodium is perceived as thirst and leads to drinking. These neurons are particularly sensitive to ethanol, responding to chronic doses as low as 40 milligrams per kilogram of body weight, with a decrease in the rate of spontaneous firing. These results were obtained from rats who had ingested ethanol for 2 to 3 weeks; normal activity did not return until 2 days after cessation of ethanol intake. Thus neurons sensitive to sodium are clearly responsive to ethanol; the mechanism might involve the direct action of ethanol on the lipids of the neuronal membrane. Other CNS neurons were shown by the same researchers to have depressed activity after chronic ingestion of ethanol in 1 gram per kilogram doses (a modest dose level for an alcoholic).

One of the frequently observed effects of ethanol ingestion is an accompanying diuresis. This increase in urine volume has been shown to be related to a suppressed secretion of vasopressin, the antidiuretic hormone (ADH). ADH is normally secreted by the supraoptic region of the posterior hypophysis. Secretion is augmented by hypertonicity, which can be brought about by increased sodium chloride intake, and diminished by hypotonicity, resulting from ingestion of a large quantity of water. Small shifts in ADH secretion occur in response to minor changes in the total concentration of salts in the blood plasma. Ethanol suppresses this regulatory secretion, leading to an increased output of water in the urine. Sodium, potassium, and chloride ions are retained. The suppressive action of ethanol on ADH occurs only while the blood ethanol concentration is rising. It diminishes in response to repeated doses.

Ethanol ingestion is also known to result in increased levels of corticosteroids in the blood plasma. The mechanism of action appears to be directed at the hypothalamus, stimulating release of the corticotropin-releasing factor (CRF), which in turn causes secretion by the pituitary of adrenocorticotropic hormone (ACTH), which then signals the adrenal cortex to secrete corticosteroids.

Thus ethanol appears to have potent actions on a "target area" consisting of parts of the hypothalamus and hypophysis, conceivably by a direct effect on neuronal membranes involving sodium transport. Possibly closely related to the effect of ethanol on sodium influx and the action potential is its effect on ATPase activity. At concentrations of ethanol no greater than 0.5%, magnesium-dependent sodium and potassium-activated ATPase activity are reduced, with a subsequent inhibition of potassium transport (see Chapter 8). Ethanol and potassium apparently compete at an allosteric site—a location on the molecule a short distance away from the primary site of action—for the association with ATPase needed to activate it. The result of the ATPase inhibition is a slowly developing partial depolarization of CNS neurons, peripheral nerve, and skeletal muscle fiber. Since amino acid transport is linked to sodium and potassium transport, the ATPase effect of ethanol might be responsible for the altered pattern of intestinal absorption referred to at the beginning of this section.

Ethanol appears to interact with several transmitters. At moderate concentrations (less than 0.2%) ethanol reduced the spontaneous release of acetylcholine from slices of rat brain cortex. However, after 22 weeks of daily ethanol ingestion rat brains had lower than normal acetylcholine concentration and lower cholinesterase concentration as well. Conceivably, a neural feedback system, responsive to the underutilized acetylcholine, led to the diminished quantities.

Ethanol also interacts with NE metabolism by inhibiting reuptake. This effect is probably due to inhibition of ATPase and the corresponding diminution of sodium and potassium gradients, since the amine pump is linked to ion flow. In human subjects ethanol altered the metabolism of NE; larger than normal quantities of reduced metabilites were produced.

Interaction with serotonin has been studied frequently. The metabolism of this transmitter in rat brain was reported to be unaffected by ethanol. It was found that preferential ingestion of ethanol by rats was augmented by infusion into the CNS ventricles of several substances, including ethanol itself and 5-hydroxy tryptophol, the reduction product arising from serotonin metabolism. Conversely, ethanol preference was reduced by prior administration of para chloro phenylalanine, an inhibitor of serotonin synthesis. When two strains of rats were bred according to ethanol preference, it was found that the strain preferring ethanol to water had higher brain serotonin and 5-HIAA than the strain preferring water. Furthermore, chronic ethanol drinking increased serotonin in the ethanol-preferring strain, but not in the water-preferring strain. Of the many studies on ethanol, these were the first to indicate a selective effect on a CNS transmitter resulting from chronic intake.

The increased basal level of serotonin, and the further increased accumulation in response to ethanol intake, clearly dependent on the genetic differences between the two strains, may provide a clue to the disease of alcoholism. Interestingly, the major change occurred in the hypothalamus which, as noted above, may be a target area for ethanol.

Chronic Ingestion of Ethanol

Alcoholic subjects have been studied extensively with a view toward identifying those biochemical and physiological changes that develop slowly during chronic ingestion of ethanol. In the course of such investigations a number of metabolic sequences were shown to be unresponsive to continued ethanol intake. Thus the serotonin content of the cerebrospinal fluid of alcoholics has been found to be within the normal range. The conversion of serotonin to 5-HIAA occurred at a normal rate, from which it was inferred that MAO and aldehyde dehydrogenase functioned normally. Similarly, the acetylcholine content of the cerebrospinal fluid of alcoholic subjects was within the normal range.

The effects of chronic ethanol intake on the alcoholic generally appear as broad changes in body chemistry. Thus, the patterns of amino acid found in the blood plasma are altered; less tryptophan, methionine, leucine, isoleucine, valine, and citrulline occur, while glutamic acid and taurine are increased. These observations are reminiscent of the experimental alterations in intestinal absorption of amino acids produced by ethanol (see above). The glutamine concentration of the blood plasma was increased when ethanol was given to normal subjects; alcoholics showed no change.

Significant changes in the electrolyte content of the whole body could be observed in alcoholics undergoing acute withdrawal. All body "spaces," including total water, extracellular water, intracellular water, and plasma volume, were increased; sodium, potassium, and chloride were present in normal concentration, and therefore occurred in increased total amount (since the total quantity is the product of the volume multiplied by the concentration). To the extent that red blood cells reflect the intracellular composition, the ionic composition of cells was altered; erythrocyte sodium was increased and potassium decreased in alcoholism.

Magnesium, a major intracellular cation, was decreased in chronic alcoholics. The plasma magnesium concentration was about 60% of normal. It is known that there is a direct effect of ethanol on the loss through excretion of the major ions; potassium and phosphate excretion is decreased while magnesium and calcium are increased. The total body magnesium content is decreased in alcoholics; the deficiency in magnesium can be reversed during a sustained alcohol-free period.

The loss of magnesium may be associated with some of the symptoms of ethanol withdrawal. Magnesium deficiency is

known to be associated with tremor, twitching, bizarre movements, convulsions, auditory and visual hallucinations, stupor,
and coma. All of these symptoms may occur during withdrawal
from ethanol; withdrawal symptoms may begin within 12 hours
after the last dose and persist for up to 10 days. It has also been
noted that patients with delerium tremens had a low erythrocyte
magnesium content.

All of the changes referred to appear to be correlated with
chronic alcohol intake; none is likely to be causally associated
with the disease of alcoholism. A faint clue may be related to the
observation that an alcohol-preferring strain of rats has an in-

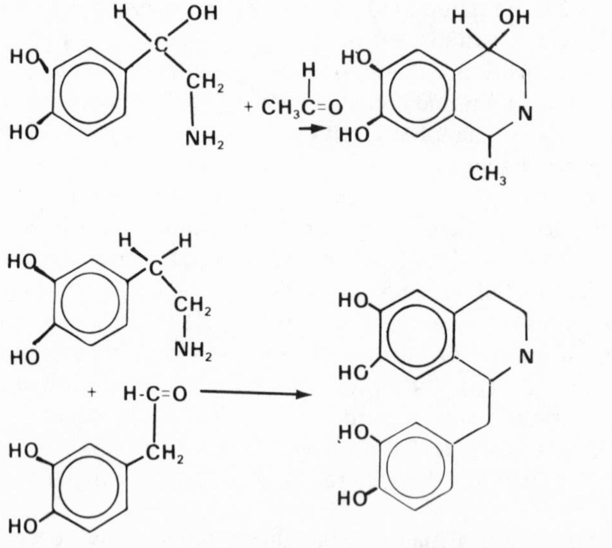

Figure 13-4. (A) the condensation of acetaldehyde with norepinephrine to produce a tetrahydroisoquinoline. (B) the condensation of
dihydroxyphenylacetaldehyde with dopamine to produce tetrahydropapaveroline.

creased CNS serotonin content (see above). The action of ethanol
on the physical structure of neuronal membranes, on the shape of
the action potential, and on ATPase may conceivably lead to

long-lasting changes in CNS organization. Recently a more specific hypothesis has been suggested. It is known that the transmitter amines readily condense with aldehydes; acetaldehyde, produced by metabolic oxidation of ethanol, is an example. The condensation product (Figure 13-4) is known as a tetrahydroisoquinoline (THIQ), and it has a structure that is similar to that of some plant alkaloids having psychopharmacological activity. It is therefore proposed that such substances, produced in excess in the CNS as a result of ethanol ingestion, might function as false transmitters, effectively disrupting the organization of the CNS. It is known that rat brain synaptosomes can accumulate such products and that a THIQ can cause the release of synaptosomal NE. A similar hypothesis proposes that in the presence of ethanol and its metabolite, acetaldehyde, the aldehyde formed from DA is metabolized more slowly and accumulated in sufficient concentration to facilitate a similar condensation. The product is tetrahydropapaveroline (Figure 13-4).

It will be apparent that at the present time there are few research leads capable of furthering the understanding and possible treatment of this crippling disease.

14

Genetic Aspects of Mental Illness

THERE IS VERY little doubt that some mental illnesses are genetically transmitted. Patterns of inheritance have been clearly shown for schizophrenia and manic-depressive disease. Earlier resistance to such findings has all but disappeared under the weight of the evidence, and current disagreements are centered around the degree of interaction of the genetic component with environmental influences. Although it might seem at first that the existence of such genetic determinants renders hopeless efforts at treatment and ultimate cure, further reflection leads to a much different viewpoint.

It is clear that genetic diseases are expressed at least in part by alterations in normal body chemistry. A genetically determined mental illness thus strongly implies altered CNS neurochemistry. Just as in the inborn chemical abnormalities of the CNS (Chapter 5), the knowledge that genetic factors are involved in a disease process leads to a more resolute search for the chemical substrates, and ultimately to the best chance of designing the most appropriate chemically based clinical management.

Genetic Transmission of Mental Illness

Determination that a disease is genetically transmitted depends upon one or more of the following lines of evidence. When the incidence of the disease is studied in the families of people who are known to be afflicted, it may be found that the proportion of cases among such families exceeds the incidence in the general population. A comparative study of the disease in pairs of monozygotic (identical) and dizygotic (fraternal) twins may show that the disease occurs more frequently in pairs of monozygotic than dizygotic twins. Finally, an analysis of the individual pedigrees of afflicted families may show an apparent pattern of transmission between generations that is consistent with simple genetic laws—a Mendelian mode of transmission.

Each of these methods, if properly applied, is theoretically capable of demonstrating genetic transmission. However, there are practical difficulties which tend to reduce the effectiveness of each method. The problems are particularly apparent when the expression of disease symptoms depends heavily upon interactions with the environment and when environmental factors alone can produce similar symptoms. The environmental factors become more than usually burdensome when diagnosis of the disease is inexact, as is presently the case with mental illnesses.

The population frequency method, as the name implies, is statistical in nature. An individual is first selected as a focus for the study, usually on the basis of a current episode of the disease. The past or current status of family members of this proband is then investigated, with respect to the disease. There are two ways to pursue the investigation. One is dependent upon recollection by the proband about other family members; this is called the family history method. The second requires clinical interviews with available family members and is called the family study method.

Difficulties in experimental design arise when the same researchers who identify and diagnose the proband also study the family for the presence of psychiatric disease; it is recognized that such a procedure is likely to produce biased results. Accordingly, in the better studies these aspects of the investigation are separated; the researchers who interview family members are unaware of the psychiatric state and diagnosis of the proband. All studies include control groups, matched for age, sex, and other relevant factors.

An increased frequency of occurrence of the disease in the families of psychiatrically ill probands is consistent with genetic transmission; however, since many families tend to share environmental factors, an additional investigative technique has been devised to sort out the environmental from the genetic factors. Recently a number of well-designed studies have focused on the comparative incidence of disease in biological and nonbiological relatives of adoptees. An increased incidence of disease in the biological relatives of ill probands is strong evidence for a genetic factor.

Data from the comparative incidence of disease in monozygotic and dizygotic twins are very useful for evaluating the possibility of genetic transmission. Although there are no two individuals who are completely identical, "identical" twins, whose genetic constitution derives from the same fertilized ovum, share most of the genetic information that is ultimately expressed in modes ranging from morphological similarity to patterns of blood enzyme activity. Thus, when comparing pairs of monozygotic and dizygotic twins, there is a greater probability that both members of a monozygotic pair will be ill if the disease has a strong genetic component. Greater concordance in monozygotic pairs has in fact been found for some mental illnesses.

In addition to the population frequency and twin study methods, which are applicable to any mode of genetic transmission, the method based on detailed pedigrees of individual families—the family tree—has also been utilized to investigate genetic transmission of mental illness. This technique requires that an identifiable disease be present in more than one generation of a particular family, with an observed pattern of illness that is consistent with either a recessive or a dominant Mendelian trait. In practice it is not likely that such results will be observed unless the disease trait is carried on a single gene, or on a cluster of contiguous genes. It is possible to sharpen the precision of this method by studying gene markers. Thus if a certain trait, such as color blindness, is known to be associated with a particular chromosome—in this case the X chromosome—then other genes on the X chromosome, located near the gene for color blindness, will be transmitted with it during the reshuffling of genetic material that accompanies multiplication of germ cells. Such an association between the marker and a gene carrying the trait for an illness, evident in particular individuals within a family, will therefore trace a pattern of genetic transmission. This association is not to be taken as causal; individuals who are color blind will not be more likely to have the disease. The association of the gene carrying the disease with the marker gene is initially random; however, once established in a given family it provides a means of tracing inheritance of the disease trait.

Schizophrenia

Evidence for a strong genetic component in schizophrenia has been accumulating since 1928, when a study of 14 pairs of monozygotic twins showed 72% concordance. A much larger study, compiled in 1946, also reported 69% concordance in 174 pairs of monozygotic twins. More recent studies find concordance rates of 40% to 50%; more rigid diagnostic criteria may be responsible for the lower concordance. A concordance rate approaching 100% would occur only if a single gene were responsible and if environmental factors had little effect on development of schizophrenic symptomatology. The observed concordance rates are consistent either with a single gene inheritance reacting with a strong environmental factor or with a polygenic mode of inheritance. In either instance the case for genetic transmission of schizophrenia is strong.

Additional evidence has recently been obtained from frequency studies among natural and adoptive kindred of schizophrenic subjects. A study was made of biological and adoptive relatives of adult schizophrenic subjects who had been adopted at an early age. Relatives of a control group of adoptees were also studied. It was found that schizophrenia or strong schizophrenic symptoms occurred in 14% of the biological relatives of the schizophrenic subjects and in 3% of their adoptive relatives. Biological relatives of control subjects had a 3% incidence and adoptive relatives had a 5.5% incidence of schizophrenia or schizophrenic symptoms. It is clear from these results that schizophrenic symptoms of adults correlate better with a genetic history of schizophrenia than with environmental factors associated with schizophrenia in the adoptive family.

Manic-Depressive Disease

It has been estimated that manic-depressive disease occurs in 1% to 3% of the general population. In contrast, 23% of the mothers and 14% of the fathers of manic-depressive patients were found to be afflicted with the same illness. It is a good inference from such findings that there is a strong genetic component to this disease. Additionally, the disproportionate distribution of the disease among male and female parents suggests that an X chromosome is involved in the transmission. The family pedigree technique has therefore become the method of choice for the study of the genetics of manic-depressive disease.

The X-transmission studies have been aided by the gene marker technique. The X chromosome is known to carry the alleles (variants of normal genes) responsible for color blindness, for the X_g blood group, and for several variants of the enzyme glucose-6-phosphate dehydrogenase (G6PD). Linkage has been reported between transmission of manic-depressive disease and both color blindness and the X_g blood group. As in all such studies, problems of diagnostic consistency vary between research groups and lend some uncertainty to the interpretation of the data.

The results to date may be summarized as follows. Although at least some instances of manic-depressive disease are transmitted via the X chromosome, some of the remaining data are consistent with autosomal (chromosomes other than X and Y) transmission; in particular several cases of apparent father-to-son transmission have been documented. Since females have an X-X chromosome pair and males have an X-Y pair in which the X chromosome is derived from the mother, father-to-son transmission is inconsistent with X-chromosome transmission.

Other studies using the population frequency and twin methods, taken together with the X-linkage data, show conclusively that at least some manic-depressive disease is genetically transmitteed.

Alcoholism

The environmental and social factors involved in the appearance of symptoms of alcoholism are large and tend to reduce the ability to demonstrate genetic factors. Nevertheless, it has been shown, largely as a result of adoptive studies, that there is a significant genetic component. Adults who were adopted in early childhood are more likely to develop alcoholism if their biological parents were alcoholic than if they are raised in an adoptive home with alcoholic foster parents.

The limited knowledge about the genetic aspects of alcoholism is at least partially related to the rather recent recognition that it is a disease, to variations in diagnostic criteria, and to the significant environmental and cultural factors involved. For example, recognized alcoholism has been reported to be five times as prevalent among men as among women; however, cultural factors make this disease much more visible among men. Such hidden diagnostic errors increase the difficulties of obtaining reliable data for genetic analysis.

Chemical Implications

The central nervous system is highly specialized with respect to its morphological structure, its overall chemical constitution, and the structured distribution of various neurochemical substances and processes within the morphological substrate. Genetic information interacts at all levels of organization with nutritional and informational input from the environment. Gross alterations in CNS function may be anticipated from a faulty mix of genetic and environmental systems at critical times during development.

Although it is usually assumed, and found, that major disturbances in CNS function with a genetic base are related to defects in enzymes or other proteins, it must be recognized that a mental illness could result from defects in organization; all of the neurochemical substances and processes may exist in normal amounts but in the wrong location. Such events, if they occur, are beyond the range of our present state of knowledge about the CNS. It is possible, however, to make some inroads into the problems deriving from faulty enzyme synthesis, as evidenced by treatments devised for the genetically based metabolic diseases outlined in Chapter 5.

The first question that arises concerns the extent to which genetic information, all of which is initially present in a single fertilized ovum, is expressed in various tissues. A method known as hybridization provides some answers. Radioactively labeled

DNA from a given tissue is mixed with an excess quantity of un-labeled RNA from the same tissue. A DNA molecule from which an RNA molecule has been transcribed will react with only that RNA molecule, and the pair can be separated from the mixture. If all of the DNA had been transcribed into RNA, then all of the radioactive DNA will hybridize (couple with) complementary RNA and 100% of the radioactivity will be removed from the mix-ture, indicating 100% utilization of the genetic information of the DNA. By this technique it is found that 10% of the genetic infor-mation is expressed in the human liver, kidney, and spleen, while 45% is expressed in the adult cerebral cortex. The figure is lower for the brainstem and for fetal brain.

Expression of genetic information thus varies from tissue to tissue, and even between different morphological entities within the CNS. Thus a given allele might be transcribed in both the cor-tex and brainstem into a variant enzyme, with varying impact upon the total pool of genetic information in each location.

It is also possible that, as a result of selective suppression, the allele may occur in one CNS location and not in others. An il-lustration of this process is provided from studies of peripheral enzymes. The enzyme G6PD exists in a number of variant forms, of which the most common is designated as G6PD-B and the next most common as G6PD-A. It has been demonstrated that in some members of a family having an AB genotype (inheritance) for G6PD, erythrocytes and leucocytes contained only G6PD-B. This selection is believed to be consistent with cloning—a process whereby an entire tissue can be derived from a single cell. The X chromosome, which contains the gene for G6PD, is present as an X-X pair in females and as an X-Y pair in males. It has been postu-lated that only one of the paired X chromosomes in females is bio-logically active and that random inactivation of one X chrom-some occurs in all cells. However, the presence of only the G6PD-B enzyme in females of the AB genotype suggested that at least in some instances the process of inactivation is selective rather than random and specific to some tissues.

One of the persistent questions in genetic research concerns experimental discrimination between three alternate models. The simplest model postulates that a disease is dependent upon the allele of a single gene. Many of the metabolic diseases described in Chapter 5 conform to this model, in which the disease is manifested when the lack of a single normal enzyme becomes critical. The critical phase may occur either during early brain development or much later in life when sudden environmental demands or stresses brought on by unrelated disease states require a level of enzyme activity that is beyond the genetically determined range.

Closely related to the single gene model is the concept of a gene cluster. The process by which sperm and ova are formed involves a reduction in the number of chromosomes, which in somatic cells are comprised of pairs of similar chromosomes, to a single chromosome representative of each pair. The representative chromosome is obtained by intermixing corresponding segments of each member of the pair, thus effectively sharing genetic information. The concept of a gene cluster assumes that several genes, whose products are critically related to a physiological function, are located so close to each other on a chromosome that they are almost always transmitted as a unit. If such a cluster is formed from alleles of the normal gene, a pronounced change in function might be expected.

One test of the cluster hypothesis was performed by measuring the relative activity of enzymes that control a particular metabolic sequence. The enzymes tyrosine hydroxylase, dopamine beta hydroxylase, and phenylethanolamine N-methyl transferase were measured in inbred strains of mice. It was found that in individual mice, activities of all three enzymes tended to vary in the same direction. As an alternative to the gene cluster hypothesis the researchers considered the possibility that one other gene, perhaps remotely located from those studied, produced a product which regulated the level of activity of the three enzymes studied. Such regulator genes are presently believed to occur frequently, along with the structural genes which synthesize enzymes and other proteins. By measuring the rate of incorporation of isotopic precursors into the three enzymes studied they found that all were synthesized at similar rates in each of the experimental animals. However, they also observed that the rate of degradation of each enzyme varied among the individual animals, thereby accounting for the observed differences in steady-state levels. They concluded that a single regulatory gene was responsible for controlling the rates of degradation of all three enzymes.

In effect, single genes and gene cluster models of inheritance are quite similar. In contrast polygenic models have different chemical implications. If alleles of two or more genes, located far apart on one chromosome or on separate chromosomes, must occur together in the same individual before a disease state is recognized, then it is highly probable that they will alter two or more metabolic sequences. For example, the possibility that deficits in both serotonin and norepinephrine metabolism must occur before manic-depressive disease is manifested (see Chapter 13) is consistent with a two-gene model for this disease.

It is therefore of considerable value to be able to identify alterations in enzymes and metabolic sequences that appear to correlate with genetic information. The enzyme MAO has been studied extensively in various clinical populations. It is known to exist as a group of closely related isoenzymes, the synthesis of each presumably being directed by a specific gene. There have been several studies of total MAO activity in blood plasma and blood platelets. One of these provided basic information, demonstrating that the enzyme activity was more closely related in monozygotic than in dizygotic twins and least of all in a random control group. From a statistical analysis of the data the researchers concluded that the hereditability, by which is meant the proportion of variance in enzyme activity between members of pairs of dizygotic twins that is due to heredity, is about 85%.

The blood platelet MAO activity was studied by another research group in pairs of monozygotic twins. One member of each pair had been diagnosed as schizophrenic. The MAO activity of both members of each pair was lower than that of normals. The researchers suggested that the reduced MAO activity might consititute a genetic marker for schizophrenia. It must be emphasized that a marker does not necessarily have a causal relation to the disease; if a gene cluster is involved the reduced MAO activity might be caused by a gene associated with the cluster, without in any way leading to schizophrenic symptomatology. Nevertheless, the association of MAO with amine metabolism, and its possible relation to dopamine, makes the report of considerable interest. Identification of the particular MAO isoenzymes present in reduced concentration would aid in the evaluation of the significance of the report because some brain MAO isoenzymes are almost specific for dopamine.

Researchers in the genetics of mental illness look to neurochemical research for knowledge about enzymes and other gene products that might serve as the gene markers which are needed to identify with certainty the patterns of inheritance. Conversely, researchers in the neurochemical aspects of mental illness would welcome a conclusive statement from the geneticists about the mode of inheritance. If one, two, or any specific number of genes are clearly shown to relate to a particular mental illness, it is clear that precisely that number of gene products are involved and remain to be identified.

But perhaps the most important conclusion from the genetic work has already been achieved. The fact that there are strong genetic components to mental illnesses demonstrates that, whether the disease is due to the right chemicals in the wrong places, to the wrong chemicals, or to too much or too little of the right chemicals, at least some mental illnesses occur only because of altered neurochemistry.

PART FOUR

An Overview

15

Some Ethical Considerations

INFORMATION AND UNDERSTANDING are the immediate objectives of all who explore natural phenomena. All researchers are aware that the knowledge obtained may contribute, directly or indirectly, to an improvement in the quality of life; many are acutely conscious of the potential for its detrimental application. But the initial search for reliable data and the synthesis of useful hypotheses occupy most of the time and effort of research scientists. "Effort" is an appropriate term; most research requires hard work, persistence against both experimental and organizational difficulties, and a willingness to commit one's time to goals that may appear illusory up until the moment that the final experiment has been completed.

The research scientist, then, is an individual possessed not only of the specialized knowledge of his field but also of a high degree of drive. He sets his own goals and chooses his own methods. To succeed at his chosen task he needs to be sure of himself and confident of his methods. Although his sense of ethics may be as high as that of his counterpart in other fields of human endeavor, it is recognized that all such people require some evaluation and feedback from others with regard to the ethical implications of their own work.

Ethical issues about an individual researcher's work are raised, then, not only by colleagues in other scientific disciplines but by people in many other fields as well. The particular circumstance that financial support for scientific research frequently derives from public or nonprofit foundation sources enhances the potency of the ethical input; disagreement over ethics is often expressed as a refusal to fund research. The validity of the ethical views expressed and enforced needs to be examined case by case; it should be expected that some will be of superior quality, many mediocre in value, and some entirely inappropriate.

With respect to biological research in general, and multidisciplinary research on brain function in particular, ethical objections have been raised concerning the use of experimental animals, the use of human subjects, and the potential danger of obtaining too much knowledge of the brain.

Animal Experimentation

Most of the research knowledge outlined in the previous chapters depends heavily upon experimentation with several species of animals ranging from mice to monkeys. Although some of the experiments involve little pain or discomfort, many are more severe. It is not possible to investigate a suspected nutritional deficiency without producing a sick animal, to investigate the potential lethality of drugs intended for human use without sometimes causing painful deaths in experimental animals, or to study detailed neural circuitry without occasionally doing major brain surgery on an animal. Some experiments are designed to be terminal; the animal is painlessly put to death at the conclusion of the experiment. Others are chronic in nature; an incapacitated animal may be kept alive for months or years.

Such procedures have been done and will be done in the pursuit of knowledge. Many people object to all animal experimentation; some choose to believe that computer simulation provides an acceptable alternative. The logic is based on the assumption that we already know so much (from previous animal experiments) that we can predict all future results by computer programming. It will be apparent from preceding chapters that we are very far from that state of knowledge in the brain sciences.

Others accept the inevitability of pain in even the best designed experiments and seek only to eliminate experiments that produce "unnecessary" pain. It is true that a few researchers throughout the history of science have chosen to carry out experiments without regard to the available and experimentally valid means for alleviating pain and discomfort in their animal subjects. Criticism by their scientific colleagues as well as by nonscientists has sometimes been effective in controlling such activities.

The instances in which communicated indignation had failed to achieve the desired control have led to massive and persistent efforts to legislate ethics. The goal is the prevention of unnecessary pain; the methods do or would include the required use of anaesthetics, which would be under conditions that could produce invalid scientific conclusions, and a heavy dependence on documentation and regulatory bodies. It is recognized that such legislation will add to the difficulties of conducting research, but it is believed that the consequent disadvantage to most researchers is necessary to properly control the unacceptable activities of a few.

I believe that the outcome will be quite different. There is no way to monitor the hour-by-hour activities of those researchers who occasionally take an ethically unacceptable shortcut and inflict unnecessary pain. Such legislation will be followed by still more restrictive legislation as occasional violations become known and arouse indignation. More restrictions on the large body of ethical researchers will eventually lead to an avoidance of research with animals. The progress of science and its benefits to all of us will diminish as a consequence of the ever-increasing severity of laws and regulations governing animal research. Some people will nevertheless feel that the legislative effort must be made and that leaving things as they are is not an acceptable alternative.

Human Experimentation

The notion that humans may be experimental subjects strikes a discordant note in all of us. We tend to feel, or hope, that, if an experiment must be done, it ought to be carried out on animals and that any procedure applied to humans should have been so well documented by prior animal research that its outcome is known beyond reasonable doubt.

The realities, of course, are much different. Experimental administration of a substance to animals gives some information about toxic dose levels and biological effects. This information, although necessary and useful in providing guidelines for subsequent application to human subjects, does not in practice lead to completely predictable results because of the substantial physiological differences between species. Particularly with respect to mental illnesses, there are no suitable animal models of illnesses such as manic-depressive disease, schizophrenia, or even alcoholism. The best that can be done is to compare the physiological and behavioral effects of a proposed new medication with the established effects of other medications known to be effective in the human disease. If the new substance is classified by such tests as a potential therapeutic agent, and if its range of toxicity in animals suggests that it will not produce serious toxicity in humans, it may then be tested in humans. Inevitably, then the initial human subjects receiving the substance are experimental subjects; research is carried out on humans. The ethics of such research has been subject to considerable debate.

The kinds of experiments related to brain function which require human subjects vary from such innocuous procedures as tests of short- and long-term retention of information and comparative studies of body metabolism in various stages of a disease process to the administration of drugs which may temporarily alter CNS function. The latter group consists of two subdivisions: those studies in which the information sought is of no immediate value to the experimental subject and those studies in which a therapeutically unproven substance is administered in the belief or hope that it will be of direct benefit to the subject. Although there is a range of ethical considerations that applies to each category, the nature of the issues is least ambiguous and is best illustrated with the last mentioned category.

Suppose that a chemical compound—let us call it Anti-S—has been tested extensively in several species of animals with the following results. In all species, no harmful effects were observed at daily dose levels less than 1 milligram of Anti-S per kilogram body weight of the test animal; at 2 milligrams per kilogram 1 of 200 experimental animals died after 6 days; at 10 milligrams per kilogram dose levels 2% of the animals died within 3 days; and at 100 milligrams per kilogram 50% of the animals died within 1 day. Furthermore, at dose levels ranging from 1 to 10 milligrams per kilogram, Anti-S altered behavior and neurophysiological parameters in a pattern similar to that of most known antischizophrenic drugs, but it appeared to be more specific than current drugs in blocking dopamine receptors, which are hypothesized to be involved in schizophrenic symptomology.

The need for better antischizophrenic drugs is real. The data for the hypothetical Anti-S would strongly suggest that it merits a trial. How does one choose the first human subject for this experiment? What dose levels will be allowed? Questions such as these are now decided by local committees on human research. Such a committee, if it allowed the initial trial, would probably require the following. The first subject is to be a medically healthy chronic schizophrenic who has not responded to any other treatment. He is to be given a dose no larger than 0.5 milligram per kilogram, and he is to be fully informed of the purpose of the experiment and its hazards. Once having volunteered to participate in the experiment, he is to be free to withdraw at any time. His consent is to be in writing and witnessed by an observer who is not a member of the research group.

It might come about that such a subject could be found and would consent to receiving Anti-S; unless he has had considerable training in a scientific discipline it is doubtful that his "informed" consent will be as meaningful as the committee hoped. Most likely the initial subject will not respond to the drug, but he will show no ill effects. The committee may then allow further tests on several similar subjects; the results will probably be the same. At this time the research group may request an increase in the allowed dose to 1 milligram per kilogram, basing their request on the observation that behavioral effects in animals were only observed at or above this dose level. Two responses are possible: the committee might reject the request on the basis that Anti-S has no proven therapeutic value and that the proposed dose is too close to the level at which an animal death occurred; or the committee might weight the "risk benefit ratio" and decide to take a chance. The risk benefit ratio is a phrase intended to mean that in any proposal involving human experimentation the sum of the benefits occurring to the patient plus those anticipated from the general increase in knowledge should outweigh the possible harm that might come to the patient. An important ethical issue therefore arises at this step. Refusal to allow an increased dose will clearly protect the next subject from any harmful effects of Anti-S. Is that choice, or the one involving further experimentation with an increased risk, the preferred ethical course?

Let us assume that the committee decided to take the risk and that further stepwise trials, each time with committee approval, with Anti-S were allowed up to a dose level of 3 milligrams per kilogram, with no patient death or serious toxicity and with some measurable improvement in 7 of 25 chronic schizophrenic subjects who were previously refractory to all other medication. At this point Anti-S would probably be regarded as a promising new drug and further tests would be projected.

Since the history of drug therapy is replete with claims of early success that are not confirmed in subsequent trials by other researchers, a scientifically valid trial of Anti-S would require a double-blind comparison with a placebo. By this procedure neither the subject nor the treating medical staff knows whether a particular subject has been given the active substance or an ineffective placebo—the assignment of the drug or placebo is made by another staff member who does not come in contact with the patients. Another widely debated ethical issue arises at this point. If Anti-S is effective, is it ethical to deprive a patient of its value by administering a placebo?

The ethical issues involved in the administration of the hypothetical Anti-S have thus included: the possible "necessary" pain involved in the preliminary animal experimentation; the question of whether any human should ever be an experimental subject; the nature of informed consent and the criteria used for choosing the first volunteer subject; the risk benefit ratio; and the placebo issue. One major issue has been left out of the discussion, and its omission reflects a lack of public concern. I have chosen to terminate the saga of Anti-S with a happy ending. It did get through the committee and had apparent value in early trials. What if the decisions had been different? The benefits of Anti-S could have been denied to many patients if the risk benefit ratio had been weighed differently.

The question here concerns the search for the "most ethical" position. Different sincere, honest, and intelligent individuals have differing ethical views. Does the public at large decide that the most ethical position is the one that imposes the most restrictions on human research? If so, Anti-S would never have been tested.

There have been some individual abuses by researchers of their responsibilities to human subjects. Doubtless a few abuses will continue to occur no matter how tightly research is regulated. But in my opinion an ethical fault occurs when beneficial research is blocked by those who appear to consider the most ethical position as the most restrictive position. There is no safe platform on which one can sit and make "objective" judgments about human conduct. And there is no safety in the view that it is always better to defer action when in doubt. Every decision, even the decision not to decide, is an action that has consequences for human affairs. A decision to reject, delay, or block a research investigation may, if it hinders needed developments, be as unethical as a decision to conduct research with unwilling subjects. Each case must be decided on the basis of extensive knowledge and general human wisdom; individuals or committees who perceive the demands of the public to be otherwise may also be held accountable for their own ethical values.

The Dangers of Knowledge

Although most of the current debate about ethics concerns human experimentation and the possible abuse of the rights of individual subjects, some people are also concerned that knowledge about brain function may soon make it possible for governments to achieve control over the behavior of whole populations.

Indeed it has been pointed out that the adult apathy resulting from malnutrition in early life does in effect provide a means of control—a government alert to this fact could perpetuate its power by manipulating the food available to infants.

The concern, however, goes much further. If there are drugs to control moods, perhaps there will soon be drugs to control learning, motivation, and social orientation. Could not such knowledge, placed into the hands of authoritarian governments, result in the perpetual subjugation of entire countries?

Although I do not believe that we are presently close to that level of knowledge, it seems to be a fair question—one that should not be answered by the shouting of political expletives. Humans' increasing understanding of nature has always resulted in the deliverance of potentially destructive power into the hands of a few. Nuclear energy is only the most recent example. Will knowledge about brain function go the same route, leaving most of us to fear the day when one all-powerful finger can not only press the nuclear button but also discharge a mind-altering aerosol throughout the world?

I think not. As I see it, all previous advances in the understanding and control of natural forces have become available to people whose brain function has been at the same operating level for thousands of years. For the first time in human history a new understanding of nature promises to change, not the world that we inhabit, but the brain in which we perceive and analyze that world. This change, if it occurs to the degree that I anticipate, will not result from a few "breakthroughs," allowing the "secret" of mind control to be delivered to malevolent people. Rather it will be a gradual process, occurring over many generations, so that each new generation will benefit from the increased knowledge about factors which optimize emotional stability and intellectual function. Such changes, if sufficiently widely disseminated, should result in humans who are better able to guard their rights and freedoms and establish wise control over the applications of new technological developments. Enlarged knowledge of the human brain, rather than constituting one more folly in human history, might provide the means for our renaissance. I see it as a goal of unquestionable ethical value.

16

Summary

THE FULL RANGE of those emotional and intellectual capabilities which we regard as uniquely human originates in an incredibly complex overlay of neurochemical organization upon highly specialized morphological structures. Not many centuries ago the possibility of knowing anything about the function of the brain seemed so hopeless that humans invented a "mind-body problem." The brain was clearly there, locked up in the skull, available for gross dissection and rudimentary analysis, but the "mind" was different—perhaps having no concrete physical location and certainly unknowable in a scientific sense.

We know better now—or we should. We do not need to mean anything more by the term mind than the total organization of functions, memories, and capabilities that characterizes any particular brain. However, although our knowledge about brain structure and function has increased dramatically in recent years, it is clear that we have progressed only a short distance toward a satisfying understanding of the nature of emotionality and thinking in mental health and illness. Our present level of understanding is sufficiently broad and sophisticated to provide the base for a rapid advance. Much of it depends upon recently acquired neurochemical data. Even at our present level of understanding it is clear that the complexity of brain organization far exceeds that of anything else we know in nature.

Organization and Growth of the Brain

The diversity of structures apparent from a study of the gross anatomy of the brain hints at its underlying complexity. Fibers interconnect brainstem regions such as the medulla and pons with the thalamus and hypothalamus, and with the cerebellum, basal ganglia, and cerebral hemispheres. Within the highly convoluted hemispheres distinct lobes are recognized and connected with each other by various association fibers. Symmetrically located regions of the two hemispheres are also linked, principally through the fibers of the corpus callosum. At the interior of the cerebral hemispheres a group of structures has been termed the limbic lobe; functional studies have related it to parts of the thalamus, hypothalamus, and the amygdaloid nucleus of the basal ganglia. The entire group has been designated as the limbic system.

Regions containing dense aggregates of neuronal cell bodies are known as nuclei. At least 25 distinct nuclei are recognized in the thalamus; some of the many functions of this region include integration and relay of sensory information, modulation of motor activity, modulation of at least that part of the electrical activity of the brain detectable in the electroencephalogram, participation with other parts of the limbic system in emotional activity, and perhaps the perception of consciousness.

Several systems of nuclei and interconnecting nerve fibers have been described. The extrapyramidal system, whose functions relate to the control of gross muscle movements, includes three of the basal ganglia, part of the subthalamus, nuclei in the midbrain known as the substantia nigra and the red nucleus, and parts of the interconnection of nuclei and short fibers in the brainstem designated as the reticular formation.

At a microscopic level there is a classification into neurons and neuroglia. Neurons, which are responsible for most or all information processing in the brain, are composed of a cell body containing many short projections known as dendrites and one large, highly branched extension known as the axon. Dendrites and the cell body receive incoming information while the axon carries the output to other neurons. The synapse, the junction between an axon and a dendrite or a cell body, is a region specialized for the chemical transmission of a nerve impulse while the axon carries the impulse as an electrochemical wave.

Neurons of several distinct sizes and shapes occur in specific locations; several layers can be recognized in the cerebral cortex and the cerebellar cortex. Classes of neuroglia include astrocytes which are interposed between blood capillaries and neurons, oligodendroglia which surround capillaries, and microglia which are apparently scavenger cells. Some neuroglia synthesize the myelin that surrounds many axons.

Within these complex morphological structures there are many specialized structural chemical entities and neurochemical processes. A large portion of the solid matter of the brain is composed of various lipids, such as cholesterol, plasmalogens, cerebrosides, sulfatides, and sphingomyelins which are associated with myelin. Other portions of the cells contain various phospholipids, fatty acids, and gangliosides. Structural proteins exist alone or in combination with lipids to form proteolipids or lipoproteins.

The brain, which requires 10% to 20% of the total energy available to the body, depends upon glycolysis and tricarboxylic acid cycle, as do other tissues. However, there is a pathway specific to the brain known as the GABA shunt, involving glutamic acid and gamma amino butyric acid. There are other biochemical pathways which are specific to the brain. The flow of nutrients, enzymes, and synthetic products occurs along the axon from the neuron cell body to the synaptic terminals. The rate of axoplasmic flow is less than 1/32 inch per day for enzymes and other proteins and as fast as 1 foot per day for amino acids, transmitter molecules, and some phospholipids. The fast rate requires energy.

Highly specialized localization of neurochemical products and processes has been demonstrated to occur within neurons.

The nucleus of a neuron contains DNA, RNA polymerase, basic proteins such as histones, and acidic proteins. Microsomes, the sites of cell synthesis found throughout the cell, have complex membranes consisting of several gangliosides and at least 16 different proteins, as well as cholesterol and phospholipids. Mitochondria, which are sites of metabolic activity, have membranes containing very little ganglioside. Mitochondrial membranes include monoamine oxidase, succinic dehydrogenase, cholinesterase, and ATPase. Half of the vitamin B_{12} found in the brain is localized in mitochondria.

There is also a highly specific regional distribution. Cell bodies of the raphe nuclei of the midbrain contain the transmitter serotonin; their axons project to three of the basal ganglia and to the thalamus and hypothalamus. These structures therefore contain the large amount of serotonin found in the synaptic terminals of the raphe nuclei. Another transmitter, dopamine, is found in other neurons of the midbrain whose axons project to the limbic system and two of the basal ganglia. Neurons of the midbrain containing norepinephrine project to the limbic system, thalamus, and hypothalamus.

The morphological and neurochemical organization of the brain, outlined above, develops and changes throughout the life of the organism. Although changes during fetal development and during the early postnatal period are the most dramatic, progressive alterations in chemical composition also occur throughout adult life. The increase in neuronal cell number that occurs prenatally is largely completed by the 7th fetal month. Axonal and dendritic growth continues past this time and myelination only begins at the 4th month postnatal. There is a critical period, occurring shortly after birth, during which certain structural and chemical growth must occur; failure to achieve the required organization at this time cannot be made up by future growth.

Brain lipids change throughout life in ways whose functional significance is not yet understood. For example, the cerebroside content of the brain is highest at 21 years, while sulfatides peak at 40 years. The proportion of lignoceric acid, a fatty acid contained in these lipids, is constant during the period 21 to 40 years, while stearic acid, another fatty acid, increases in cerebrosides but not in sulfatides. Other examples of detailed changes in structural chemistry are known. Simpler substances also change with age. Thus the iron content of the thalamus peaks at age 30, while the peak age is 50 in the putamen, one of the basal ganglia. In contrast other substances, such as the S-100 brain-specific protein, increase throughout life, while still others, such as the enzyme glucose-6-phosphate dehydrogenase, are constant throughout life.

At least some of the changes in neurochemical composition are dependent upon adequate nutrition. Malnutrition results in a decrease in neurons and neuroglia, with a concomitant decrease in myelin lipids and in gangliosides and phospholipids. Some of the effects of malnutrition occurring during the first 2 years of life are irreversible. Growth of neurons and myelinated interconnections cannot be restored by subsequent adequate nutrition. An atypical myelin may also be formed. Behavioral consequences include mental retardation in severe cases and apathy in less severe cases.

The brain is acutely dependent upon adequate nutrition throughout life. For example, a total lack of vitamin B_1 for a few days has been reported to lead to lassitude, irritability, and anorexia; niacin deficits are accompanied by depression, hallucinations, and other mental symptoms before the appearance of the characteristic symptoms of pellagra; and B_{12} deficiencies lead to memory loss as well as other symptoms.

There is a formal correspondence of the effects on brain development between malnutrition and the genetic metabolic diseases. Each deprives the brain of metabolites needed for growth and each can result in mental retardation or other severe symptoms if the deficiency occurs during the critical period. The genetic diseases, because they are each caused by the lack of a single enzyme, have more specific symptomatology. Some of these diseases are recognized to occur as either infantile or juvenile forms; occasionally an adult variation is recognized. For example, Nieman-Pick disease, in which sphingomyelin accumulates because of a lack of the enzyme sphingomyelinase, generally occurs in infancy, with symptoms including slow psychomotor development, ataxia, tremor and convulsions, and death by age 3. In some cases the same enzyme deficit does not become manifest until ages 1 to 5; survival usually extends into adolescence. When the first symptoms appear after the age of 5 and survival into adult life occurs, emotional and thought disturbances precede the more concrete symptoms. Similarly in metachromatic leukodystrophy, a disease due to the deficiency of the enzyme cerebroside sulfatase accompanied by an increase in sulfatides and an abnormal myelin, symptoms in the less frequent adult form may begin with depression and schizoid behavior. Again in the juvenile form of Tay-Sachs disease the early symptoms include personality changes and a progressive psychosis. This disease is caused by an accumulation of a monosialoganglioside and is characterized by a lack of the enzyme hexosaminidase-A.

Genetic diseases of amino acid metabolism, such as phenylketonuria and leucinosis, are accompanied by mental retardation unless treatment is instituted shortly after birth. An inability to metabolize the amino acid phenylalanine leads to a great increase in its concentration in the blood, where it competes with other amino acids for entry into the brain. The brain thus becomes nutritionally deficient in the balanced mixture of amino acids needed for protein synthesis and mental retardation results, just as when protein undernutrition occurs. One variant of leucinosis provides just enough enzyme for normal function until the patient is stressed by infections or other illnesses; disease symptoms then rapidly occur.

Not all genetic diseases are caused by enzyme deficiencies. There are genetic disorders of vitamin B_{12} metabolism which are caused by deficiencies in proteins required to absorb it from the intestine into the bloodstream. The resulting deficiency leads to mental retardation, cerebellar and spinal cord dysfunction, and early death.

The changes in brain development because of nutritional or genetic deficiencies that occur during the critical period are not unexpected, considering our current state of knowledge. In contrast, the phenomenon described as chemical imprinting could not have been predicted from previous knowledge. It has recently been found that the transient presence of a particular substance shortly after birth will permanently alter the adult behavior of experimental animals. Thus, normal male or female sexual behavior in rats is grossly disturbed by the administration of estrogens shortly after birth; female rats become sexually unreceptive as adults, and male rats, when adult, are unable to ejaculate and show misdirected mounting of females. In addition the normal estrous cycle of the female never develops. It has been shown that a portion of the hypothalamus that is normally organized so as to produce cyclic changes becomes acyclic as a result of the presence of estrogen during the critical period.

Similarly, diurnal variations in corticosteroid secretion, also dependent upon hypothalamic control in the adult, never appear if corticosteroids are present during the critical period. Details of the mechanisms of such organizational changes are presently under intense investigation; success in this field is likely to lead to powerful new insights into brain organization.

Information Processing

The brain receives, stores, processes, and transmits information. It is useful, and perhaps mandatory, that any attempt to understand brain function should take into account some of the elements of information theory. The apparent all-or-none nature of the nerve impulse led to early attempts to model the brain as a complex array of binary elements. Logical nets had been constructed of two-state switches and shown to possess decision-making capability—so-called "artificial intelligence." These efforts were paralleled by the conceptualization of neural models which were intended to produce reliable responses. One class of models achieved this goal on the basis of deterministic organization; another was based on probabilistic organization and required redundancy to achieve reliability.

A model of the function of the cerebellar cortex, based on probabilistic concepts and on data about the observed neural interconnections, was claimed to be consistent with the observed function of this region. A deterministic model of the olfactory system of the cat, also based on known neuroanatomy, was also said to be consistent with biological function. Information processing was also studied by observing the details of neural organization in the eye. It was shown that lateral inhibition of nearby receptor cells provided a mechanism for sharpening information. A more extensive study of neural organization described the interconnected striatal circuits that control extrapyramidal function.

The process by which the brain transmits information between neurons consists of three components: the action potential, synaptic transmission, and postsynaptic response. The action potential arises as a result of a sudden change in the resting potential across nerve membranes. The resting potential is dependent upon an energy-requiring "pump" that accumulates potassium ions and excludes sodium ions within the cell, and also upon a membrane that in the resting state is somewhat permeable to potassium and only very slightly permeable to sodium. The result is a potential difference of 50 to 100 millivolts across the membrane, with the interior being negatively charged. A brief reversal of this permeability condition can occur at any point along the axon and constitutes an action potential. Adjacent regions are then stimulated and a wave travels down the axon.

At the synapse this electrochemical wave leads to the release of specific transmitter molecules which move across the junction and set in motion events which depolarize or hyperpolarize the postsynaptic membrane. Successive depolarizations eventually lead to generation of an action potential by the target neuron; hyperpolarization reduces the possibility that this will occur. There are presently four known substances as well as an additional five substances believed to have transmitter activity. Each of these in effect carries an individual message signaling to the target neuron the kind of cell with which it is in communication.

Brain function also requires the capability of information storage. Memory mechanisms are presently being researched. It would seem, from the vast amount of information presumed to be stored in memory, that storage in patterned molecules is the only mode which can accomodate the required quantity. Accordingly, much effort has been devoted to a search for "memory molecules." The storage of genetic information in RNA provides an attractive model to some. Others lean toward proteins or peptides.

Evidence that RNA or proteins are involved in memory storage comes from studies of retrograde amnesia. It is possible to train an animal to perform a task prior to injecting it with a protein or RNA synthesis inhibitor and then to observe that memory fails in that animal and not in a noninjected control. Thus consolidation of memory, or formation of long-term memory, is thought to require RNA or protein synthesis; it is also thought that it is possibly located in some of the molecules synthesized. Similarly, retrieval of memory may also be dependent upon concurrent synthesis of RNA or protein.

The act of learning is distinguished from the formation of memory by the concept of insight. It can be shown that experimental animals can assemble elements of information presented to them and then use those elements to perform a task successfully. This assembly process, and not the subsequent retention of the required performance, requires an increased rate of RNA synthesis in the limbic system.

Chemistry and Uncontrolled Behavior

The highly complex morphological and neurochemical organization of the brain is a necessary condition for its ability to process a wide range of information. Precisely timed and organized feedback systems keep brain function within a biologically desirable range. Their precision and complexity are developed in conjunction with a means to hold variations in the chemical environment within narrow limits. When these limits are exceeded, as by the ingestion of some substances or by genetically based failures in the internal regulatory mechanisms, uncontrolled behavior results.

Amphetamine, in small doses, reduces appetite and induces insomnia. Larger doses produce a psychotic state which is considered by some to be strikingly similar to schizophrenic psychoses. Several neurochemical studies implicate the transmitter dopamine as central to the amphetamine psychosis and to the stereotyped behavior that frequently accompanies it. Amphetamine also produces psychomotor activation, apparently because of its effect on norepinephrine-containing neurons. Its effect on sleep may be due to interaction with serotonin-containing neurons. It is apparent, then, that amphetamine can disrupt at least three transmitter systems.

LSD is a most potent psychotomimetic substance, apparently producing behavioral effects in doses so low that less than 10 molecules would be present at each synapse. The central characteristics of the LSD effect can be described as a scrambling of information processing; sensory input appears to fluctuate in intensity, sensory modalities overlap each other's domain, and a loss of temporal relations implies a disorganization of short-term memory. The low effective dose and the profound disruption suggest that LSD targets on some neural systems responsible for sequencing information flow in the entire brain. There is some evidence that LSD reduces the utilization of serotonin and blocks the spontaneous activity of all of the serotonin-containing raphe nuclei. It is not clear at present whether this is its primary target area.

Drugs such as atropine, scopolamine, and the piperidyl benzilate esters block receptors which are normally stimulated by the transmitter acetylcholine. In large doses a "toxic delirium" results; the experience is described as frightening and includes auditory hallucinations, paranoia, and a retrograde amnesia.

The experience of mood change is common to all of us. It is believed that the changes in affective state that characterize manic-depressive disease are an intensification of normal variations in mood. A hypothesis, developed over the past 15 years, relates mood levels to the amount of amine transmitter available for functional use at the synaptic junction. Intensive research investigations have succeeded in detailing the neurochemical mechanisms that control the synthesis and metabolism of these transmitters. Synthesis occurs under the influence of enzymes whose activity can be regulated, in a biochemical negative feedback loop, by the synthetic products. Other enzymes, such as monoamine oxidase (MAO), impose a further regulation on amine concentrations by metabolizing them to inactive products. Inhibitors of MAO, when given to animals, produce a behavioral excitation.

Mood is affected not only by regulators of amine synthesis but by the steroid hormones as well. One of these, progesterone, appears to be associated with premenstrual depression. In some instances the steroid hormones appear to act on amine transmitter availability; for example, corticosterone activates an amine pump which is responsible for the reaccumulation of norepinephrine in the presynaptic regions.

Severe disturbances in affect characterize manic-depressive disease. Hopelessness, low self-esteem, guilt, and suicidal ideation are common symptoms of depression, while pressured speech, racing thoughts, and grandiosity occur frequently during hypomanic episodes. The amine hypothesis of affective state arose after it was noted that the use of reserpine was frequently accompanied by depression and that reserpine lowered brain serotonin in experimental animals, while iproniazid, which inhibits MAO, produced a behavioral excitation.

Antidepressant drugs were developed in conformity with this hypothesis. Inhibitors of MAO, as well as a group of substances known as tricyclic antidepressants, which inhibit the reuptake of transmitter amines from the synaptic cleft, have been useful in treating many depressions.

Antimanic drugs include the potent antipsychotic agents, such as fluphenazine; this substance has been shown to inhibit a variant of the enzyme adenyl cyclase that occurs in the striatum. This particular enzyme is activated by the transmitter dopamine; by its action it promotes the formation of cyclic AMP. This latter substance has been postulated to trigger permeability changes in the postsynaptic membrane. Thus the system dopamine—adenyl cyclase—cyclic AMP is part of the chain of transmission of information between neurons. Inhibition by fluphenazine would block the sequence and slow down neural information processing, presumably leading to a state of reduced behavioral activity.

The antipsychotic agents are nonspecific and may produce unacceptable dampening of behavior when used to treat mania. In contrast lithium is specific and effective in the therapy of mania as well as in some instances in the prophylaxis of manic-depressive disease. Some of the neurochemical effects of lithium support the amine hypothesis; it reduces the functional utilization of the amine transmitters. However, it also acts directly on isolated nerves to shorten the action potential, decreases nerve conduction velocity, and alters the activity of the enzyme ATPase, which is part of the pump mechanism that removes sodium from intracellular fluid. Another simple ion, rubidium, has many effects which may be termed "opposite" to those of lithium, and it is currently being tested for antidepressant activity. It is possible that lithium and rubidium may both act primarily on axonal membranes to alter the energy of the action potential.

Schizophrenic symptomatology is presently believed to be expressed through dopamine systems. The evidence is inferential, based in part on the relation of amphetamine to dopamine and the concomitant amphetamine psychosis and partly on the fact that the most potent drugs for alleviation of schizophrenic symptoms have extrapyramidal and therefore dopamine-linked side effects. Additionally, it has been claimed that the enzyme dopamine beta hydroxylase, which converts dopamine to norepinephrine, is lower than normal in parts of the schizophrenic brain.

Alcoholism, another major mental illness, has not yet been studied in as great detail as manic-depressive disease and schizophrenia. It is known, however, that ethanol alters neural membranes, reduces ATPase activity, and has at least the hypothalamus as one of its target regions. Chronic ethanol intake profoundly changes body electrolyte composition, increasing potassium and phosphate and decreasing magnesium and calcium content.

The postulate that manic-depressive disease and schizophrenia are causally related to neurochemical factors is strengthened considerably by evidence for a strong genetic factor in the disease process. Concordance rates in monozygotic twins and studies of the foster families and natural families of schizophrenic subjects who had been adopted in childhood make it clear that inherited factors are important in the development of schizophrenic symptomatology. Similarly, population frequency studies, twin studies, and family pedigree studies all point clearly to a strong genetic factor in manic-depressive disease. With alcoholism there is also clear evidence for a genetic predisposition, although environmental factors are strong; a chemical basis for alcoholism is therefore likely.

To date it has not been possible to determine whether a single gene or several genes are involved in each of these diseases. There is some evidence, however, that in at least some instances of manic-depressive disease genetic transmission may occur via a dominant gene on the X chromosome. In these cases, then, a search for a single faulty gene product, presumably either an abnormal enzyme or a deformed protein, has some hope of meeting with success.

It is clear, in review, that a multiplicity of brain functions, from control of gross motor movements to sensitive alterations in mood, are dependent upon the neurochemical integrity of the brain. Particularly during the critical period of brain development, deficiencies in nutrition and alterations in the internal chemical environment and in genetically based regulatory machanisms are likely to produce significant perturbations of brain organization. Some of these may appear only much later in life as profound behavioral disturbances. Additionally, since chemical changes in the brain occur throughout life, alteration in the chemical environment at any time ay have behavioral consequences.

These conclusions are reasonable even with the limited knowledge we now possess. We can expect more detailed and useful insights in the not too distant future, as scientists, building on the present base, rapidly research some of the currently unanswered questions and formulate more specific hypotheses.

Much of the knowledge already obtained as well as some of that still to be gained has depended upon research with human subjects. The ethics of such research procedures are currently subject to a variety of challenges and defenses from equally sincere people. Future research will necessarily be guided by an ethical consensus; provided that the consensus is not heavily weighted by the deceptive safety of overrestriction, it is possible that the knowledge gained in this field may be applied to improve the quality of human emotional and intellectual performance.

Suggestions for Further Reading

1. Bossy, Jean. Atlas of Neuroanatomy and Special Sense Organs. Philadelphia, W. B. Saunders Co., 1970.

2. Bourne, Geoffrey H., ed. The Structure and Function of Nervous Tissue, Vol. II. New York, Academic Press, 1969.

3. Bowman, Robert E., and Dalla, Sarinda P., eds. Biochemistry of Brain and Behavior. New York, Plenum Press, 1972.

4. Brazier, Mary A. B., Waller, Donald O., and Schneider, Diana, eds. Neural Modeling. Los Angeles, Brain Research Institute, University of California, 1973.

5. Byrne, William L., ed. Molecular Approaches to Learning and Memory. New York, Academic Press, 1970.

6. Efron, Daniel H., ed. Psychotomimetic Drugs. New York, Raven Press, 1970.

7. Ehrenpreis, Seymour, and Solnitzky, Othmar, eds. Neurosciences Research, Vol. I. New York, Adademic Press, 1968.

8. Essman, Walter B., and Valzelli, L., eds. Current Developments in Psychopharmacology. New York, Spectrum Publications, 1975.

9. Feigenbaum, E. A., and Feldman, J., eds. Computers and Thought. New York, McGraw-Hill, 1963.

10. Fieve, Ronald R., Rosenthal, David, and Brill, Henry, eds. Genetic Research in Psychiatry. Baltimore, The Johns Hopkins University Press, 1975.

11. Gaull, Gerald E., ed. Biology of Brain Dysfunction, 2 vols. New York, Plenum Press, 1973.

12. Hamburg, Max, and Barrington, E. J. W., eds. Hormones in Development. New York, Appleton-Century-Crofts, 1971.

13. Himwich, Williamina H., and Himwich, Harold E., eds. Progress in Brain Research, Vol. 9, The Developing Brain. New York, Elsevier Publishing Co., 1964.

14. Ho, Beng T., and McIsaac, William M., eds. Brain Chemistry and Mental Disease, New York, Plenum Press, 1971.

15. Hoffer, A., and Osmond, H. The Hallucinogens. New York, Academic Press, 1967.

16. Hommes, F. A., and Van den Berg, C. J. Inborn Errors of Metabolism. New York, Academic Press, 1973.

17. Kissin, Benjamin, and Begleiter, Henri, eds. The Biology of Alcoholism, Vol. I, Biochemistry. New York, Plenum Press, 1971.

18. Lajtha, Abel, ed. Handbook of Neurochemistry, Vol. I, Chemical Architecture of the Nervous System. New York, Plenum Press, 1969.

19. Lajtha, Abel, ed. Handbook of Neurochemistry, Vol. VI, Alteration of Chemical Equilibrium in the Nervous System. New York, Plenum Press, 1971.

20. Lajtha, Abel, ed. Handbook of Neurochemistry, Vol. VII, Pathological Chemistry of the Nervous System, New York, Plenum Press, 1972.

21. Lajtha, Abel, and Ford, D. H., eds. Progress in Brain Research, Vol. 29, Brain Barrier Systems. New York, Elsevier Publishing Co., 1968.

22. Levine, Seymour, ed. Hormones and Behavior. New York, Academic Press, 1972.

23. Lissak, K., ed. Hormones and Brain Function. New York, Plenum Press, 1973.

24. Mandell, Arnold J., ed. New Concepts in Neurotransmitter Regulation. New York, Plenum Press, 1973.

25. McGaugh, James L., ed. The Chemistry of Mood, Motivation, and Memory. New York, Plenum Press, 1972.

26. McIlwain, Henry, and Bachelord, H. S. Biochemistry and the Central Nervous System, 4th edition: Edinburgh, Churchhill Livingstone, 1971.

27. Michael, Richard P., ed. Endocrinology and Human Behavior. London, Oxford University Press, 1968.

28. Pappas, George, and Purpura, Dominick P., eds. Structure and Function of Synapses. New York, Raven Press, 1972.

29. Pfeiffer, Carl C., and Smythies, John R., eds. International Review of Neurobiology, Vol. 13. New York, Academic Press, 1970.

30. Purpura, Dominick, and Schade, J. P., eds. Progress in Brain Research, Vol. 4, Growth and Maturation of the Brain. New York, Elsevier Publishing Co., 1964.

31. Rech, Richard H., and Moore, Kenneth E., eds. Introduction to Psychopharmacology. New York, Raven Press, 1971.

32. Sabelli, Hector C., ed. Chemical Modulation of Brain Function. New York, Raven Press, 1973.

33. Schmitt, Francis O., and Worden, Frederic G., eds. The Neurosciences: Third Study Program. Cambridge, Mass., The MIT Press, 1974.

34. Seixas, Frank H., and Eggleston, Suzie, eds. Alcoholism and the Central Nervous System. Annales of the New York Academy of Sciences, Vol. 215, 1973.

35. Shader, Richard I., ed. Psychiatric Complications of Medical Drugs. New York, Raven Press, 1972.

36. Scrimshaw, Nevin S., and Gordon, John E., eds. Malnutrition, Learning, and Behavior. Cambridge, Mass, The MIT Press, 1968.

37. Stevens, Charles F. Neurophysiology: A Primer. New York, John Wiley and Sons, 1966.

38. Talland, George H., and Waugh, M. C., eds. The Pathology of Memory. New York, Academic Press, 1969.

39. Thompson, Travis, and Schuster, Charles R. Behavioral Pharmacology. Englewood Cliffs, N. J., Prentice-Hall, 1968.

40. Truex, Raymond C. Strong and Elwyn's Human Neuroanatomy, 4th edition. Baltimore, The Williams and Wilkins Co., 1959.

41. Von Neumann, J. The Computer and the Brain. New Haven, Conn., Yale University Press, 1958.

42. Wallaas, Otto, ed. Molecular Basis of Some Aspects of Mental Activity, Vol. 1. New York, Academic Press, 1966.

The following articles, appearing in the books listed above, have particular relevance to some of the chapters in this book.

Chapter 1
Bodian, David. Synaptic diversity and characterization by electron microscopy (in 28).
Chapter 2
Rouser, George, and Yamamoto, Akira. Lipids. (in 18).
Folch-Pi, Jordi. The composition of nervous membranes (in 21).
Chapter 3
Dobbing, John. The development of the blood-brain barrier (in 21).
Horwitt, M. K. Effect of diet on lipid composition of brain (in 13).
LaValle, A. Critical periods of neuronal maturation (in 13).
Chapter 4
Winick, Myron, and Rosso, Pedro. Effects of malnutrition on brain development (in 11).
Chapter 5
Bickel, H. The clinical pattern of inborn metabolic errors with brain damage (in 16).
Brady, Roscoe O. Lipidoses (in 20).
Kalckar, H. M., Kenoshita, J. H., and Donnel, G. N. Galactosemia: biochemistry, genetics, pathophysiology, and developmental aspects (in 11).

Nyhan, William C. Disorders of nucleic acid metabolism (in 11).

Rosenberg, L. E., and Mahoney, M. J. Inherited disorders of methyl-malonate and vitamin B metabolism. A progress report (in 16).

Suzuki, Kunihiko, and Suzuki, Kinuko. Disorders of sphingolipid metabolism (in 11).

Chapter 6

Balazs, R. Effects of disturbing metabolic balance, in the early postnatal period, on brain development (in 16).

Krieger, Dorothy T. Pathophysiology of central nervous system regulation of anterior pituitary function (in 11).

McEwen, Bruce S., Zigmond, Richard, Azmitior, Efron C., Jr., and Weiss, Jay W. Steroid hormone interactions with specific brain regions (in 3).

Woodbury, Dixon M. Biochemical effects of adrenocorticosteroids on the central nervous system (in 20).

Chapter 7

Barbeau, Andre. Biology of the striatum (in 11).

Cowan, Jack. The design of reliable systems (in 4).

Freeman, Walter. A model of the olfactory system (in 4).

Hunt, E. B. Programming a model of concept for mation (in 9).

Turing, H. M. Computing machinery and intelligence (in 9).

Chapter 8

Grundfest, Harry. Synaptic and ephaptic transmission (in 2).

Chapter 9

Barondes, Samuel H., and Squire, L. R. Slow biological processes in memory storage and "recovery" of memory (in 25).

Deutch, J. Anthony. The cholinergic synapse and the site of memory (in 25).

Essman, Walter B. Purine metabolism in memory consolidation (in 5).

Glassman, E., and Wilson, J. E. The effect of short experiences on macromolecules in the brain (in 3).

Hyden, Holger, and Lange, Paul W. Correlation of the S-100 brain protein with behavior (in 3).

McConnell, J.V., Shigehesa, T., and Saliv, H. Attempts to transfer approach and avoidance responses by RNA injections in rats (in 5).

Chapter 10

Barondes, Samuel H. Some critical variables in studies of the effects of inhibition of protein synthesis on memory (in 5).

Bowman, R. E., and Kottler, Paul D. Regional brain RNA metabolism as a function of different experiences (in 3).

Jarvick, Murray E. The role of consolidation in memory (in 5).

Chapter 11

Abood, Leo G. Stereochemical and membrane studies with the psychotomimetic glycolate esters (in 6).

Angrist, Burton M., and Gershon, Samuel. Psychiatric sequelae of amphetamine use (in 35).

Griffith, J. D., Cavanaugh, J. H., and Oats, M. D. Psychosis induced

by the administration of d-amphetamine to human volunteers (in 6).
Shader, Richard I., and Greenblatt, David J. Belladonna alkaloids and synthetic anticholinergics. Uses and toxicity (in 35).
Snyder, Solomon H., Weingartner, Herbert, and Faillace, Louis A. DOET (2, 5-dimethoxy-4-ethylamphetamine) and DOM (STP) (2, 5, dimethoxy-4-methylamphetamine), new psychotropic agents: their effects in man (in 6).
Stein. Larry, and Wise, C. David. Mechanism of the facilitating effects of amphetamine on behavior (in 6).
Sulser, Fredolin, and Sanders-Bush, Elaine. Biochemical and metabolic considerations concerning the mechanism of action of amphetamine and related compounds (in 6).

Chapter 12

Alivisatos, S. G. A., and Tabakoff, B. Formation and metabolism of "biogenic" aldehydes (in 32).
Axelrod, Julius. Regulation of the neurotransmitter norepinephrine (in 33).
Bloom, Floyd L., Hoffer, Barry J., and Siggins, George R. Central noradrenergic receptors: localization, function, and molecular mechanisms (in 24).
Dairman, Wallace. Multiple measures of compensation in catecholamine biosynthesis (in 24).
Glick, Ira D., and Bennet, Susan E. Psychiatric effects of progesterone and oral contraceptives (in 35).
Glowinski, Jacques, Hamon, Michel, and Hery, Francis. Regulation of serotonin synthesis in central serotoninergic neurons (in 24).
Iverson, Leslie C. Biochemical aspects of synaptic modulation (in 33).
Kety, Seymour. Brain amines and affective disorders (in 14).
Maas, James W. Interactions between adrenocortical steroid hormones, electrolytes, and the catecholamines (in 14).
Prange, Arthur J., Jr., and Lipton, Morris H. Hormones and behavior: some principles and findings (in 35).
Rose, Robert M. The psychological effects of androgens and estrogens (in 35).
Sabelli, H. C., and Giardina, W. J. Amine modulation of affective behavior (in 32).
Ungerstedt, Urban. Functional dynamics of central monoamine pathways (in 33).

Chapter 13

Anton, F., Eccleston, D., and Smythies, J. P. Transmethylation processes in schizophrenia (in 14).
Cohen, Gerald. Tetrahydroisoquinoline alkaloids: uptake, storage, and secretion by the adrendal medulla and by adrenergic neurons (in 34).
Curzon, G. Relationships between stress and brain serotonin and their possible significance in affective disorders (in 14).
Flink, Edmund B. Mineral metabolism in alcoholism (in 17).

Greenberg, R. N, N-dimethylated and N, N-diethylated indole-amines in schizophrenia (in 32).

Hollister, Leo E. Chemotherapy of schizophrenia (in 14).

Kalant, Harold. Absorption, diffusion, distribution, and elimination of ethanol: effects on biological membranes (in 17).

Meltzer, Herbert L., and Fieve, Ronald R. Rubidium in psychiatry and medicine: an overview (in 8).

Mendelson, Jack H. Biochemical mechanisms of alcohol addiction (in 17).

Poser, Charles M. Demyelination in the central nervous system in chronic alcoholism: central pontine myelinolysis and Marchiafava-Bignami's disease (in 34).

Wayner, Matthew J. Effects of ethyl alcohol on lateral hypothalamic neurons (in 34).

Chapter 14

Fieve, Ronald R., Mendlewicz, Julien, Rainer, John D., and Fleiss, Joseph. A dominanat X-linked factor in manic-depressive illness (in 10).

Motulsky, Arno G., and Omenn, Gilbert S. Biochemical genetics and psychiatry (in 10).

The data of Tables 3-1, 3-2, and 3-3 were recalculated from Rouser and Yamamoto (in 18).

INDEX

Herbert L. Meltzer, Ph.D., received his doctorate from Columbia University and has served as a research scientist in neurochemistry at the New York Psychiatric Institute since 1950.

Dr. Meltzer has published work in several distinguished professional journals, concentrating his studies on the application of neurochemical findings to clinical research.

Date Due